Approaches to Measuring
Human Behavior
in the Social Environment

Approaches to Measuring Human Behavior in the Social Environment has been co-published simultaneously as *Journal of Human Behavior in the Social Environment*, Volume 11, Numbers 3/4 2005.

Approaches to Measuring Human Behavior in the Social Environment

William R. Nugent, PhD
Editor

Approaches to Measuring Human Behavior in the Social Environment has been co-published simultaneously as *Journal of Human Behavior in the Social Environment*, Volume 11, Numbers 3/4 2005.

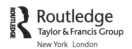

Routledge
Taylor & Francis Group
New York London

First published by

The Haworth Social Work Practice Press, 10 Alice Street, Binghamton, NY 13904-1580 USA

The Haworth Social Work Practice Press is an imprint of The Haworth Press, Inc., 10 Alice Street, Binghamton, NY 13904-1580 USA.

This edition published 2012 by Routledge

Routledge	Routledge
Taylor & Francis Group	Taylor & Francis Group
711 Third Avenue	2 Park Square, Milton Park
New York, NY 10017	Abingdon, Oxon OX14 4RN

Approaches to Measuring Human Behavior in the Social Environment has been co-published simultaneously as *Journal of Human Behavior in the Social Environment*, Volume 11, Numbers 3/4 2005.

Cover design by Kerry Mack

Library of Congress Cataloging-in-Publication Data

Approaches to measuring human behavior in the social environment/William R. Nugent, editor.
    p. cm.
    "Co-published simultaneously as Journal of human behavior in the social environment, volume 11, numbers 3 and 4, 2005."
    Includes bibliographical references and index.
    ISBN-13: 978-0-7890-3082-5 (hard cover: alk. paper)
    ISBN-10: 0-7890-3082-9 (hard cover: alk. paper)
    ISBN-13: 978-0-7890-3083-2 (soft cover: alk. paper)
    ISBN-10: 0-7890-3083-7 (soft cover: alk. paper)
    1. Psychometrics. 2. Human behavior. 3. Social psychology. I. Nugent, William R.
BF39.A67 2005
302–dc22   2005016218

Approaches to Measuring Human Behavior in the Social Environment

CONTENTS

ABOUT THE EDITOR

William R. Nugent, PhD, is Professor and Director of the PhD Program in the College of Social Work at the University of Tennessee. He previously taught at the University of Maryland at Baltimore, Florida International University, and Florida State University. He has also worked as an outpatient psychotherapist, as a counselor for the hearing-impaired, and as training coordinator for a network of family service agencies and runaway shelters. Dr. Nugent has published over 50 articles in peer-reviewed journal and is a co-author, with Dr. Jackie Sieppert and Dr. Walter Hudson, of the recently published *Practice Evaluation in the 21st Century*. He has conducted research on measurement and assessment methods, adolescent antisocial behavior, victim-offender mediation, and intervention outcomes.

Psychometric Evaluation
of the Structured Clinical Interview
for DSM-IV Childhood Diagnoses
(KID-SCID)

Douglas C. Smith
Diane L. Huber
James A. Hall

SUMMARY. The purpose of this study was to evaluate the reliability and validity of selected modules of the Structured Clinical Interview for DSM-IV (KID-SCID, Version 1.0). The Disruptive Behavior Disorders (i.e., ADHD, ODD, CD) and Substance Related Disorders modules of the KID-SCID were administered to 50 adolescents receiving residential treatment for substance abuse and severe behavioral problems. This study examined available evidence for inter-rater reliability and conver-

Douglas C. Smith, MSW, LMSW, is SCY Program Coordinator, Adolescent Health and Resource Center, Iowa City, IA.

Diane L. Huber, PhD, is Professor in Nursing, University of Iowa. James A. Hall, PhD, is Professor in Pediatrics, Social Work and Public Health, University of Iowa.

Address correspondence to: Douglas C. Smith, MSW, LMSW, SCY Program Coordinator, Adolescent Health and Resource Center, 509 Kirkwood Avenue, Iowa City, IA 52240 (E-mail: douglas-c-smith@uiowa.edu).

This article was supported by a grant from the University of Iowa Obermann Center for Advanced Studies Spelman Rockefeller Grant Program (CASSPR), D. Huber, PI.

[Haworth co-indexing entry note]: "Psychometric Evaluation of the Structured Clinical Interview for DSM-IV Childhood Diagnoses (KID-SCID)." Smith, Douglas C., Diane L. Huber, and James A. Hall. Co-published simultaneously in *Journal of Human Behavior in the Social Environment* (The Haworth Social Work Practice Press, an imprint of The Haworth Press, Inc.) Vol. 11, No. 3/4, 2005, pp. 1-21; and: *Approaches to Measuring Human Behavior in the Social Environment* (ed: William R. Nugent) The Haworth Social Work Practice Press, an imprint of The Haworth Press, Inc., 2005, pp. 1-21. Single or multiple copies of this article are available for a fee from The Haworth Document Delivery Service [1-800-HAWORTH, 9:00 a.m. - 5:00 p.m. (EST). E-mail address: docdelivery@haworthpress.com].

gent validity. Convergent validity was demonstrated for the Disruptive Behavior Disorders module, however, the Substance Abuse Disorders module failed to converge with frequency of use for most substances. Inter-rater reliability was generally high. This research provides initial evidence for both the reliability and validity of the Disruptive Behavior and Substance Abuse Disorders modules of the KID-SCID, making these modules useful in clinical practice with adolescents in treatment for substance abuse and conduct disorder. *[Article copies available for a fee from The Haworth Document Delivery Service: 1-800-HAWORTH. E-mail address: <docdelivery@haworthpress.com> Website: <http://www.HaworthPress.com> © 2005 by The Haworth Press, Inc. All rights reserved.]*

KEYWORDS. Substance abuse, adolescence, psychometric testing, research

Social workers should benefit from reliable and valid measures of both substance abuse and antisocial behaviors among adolescents. Perhaps the most compelling reason for such measures is simply that social workers are likely to encounter adolescents with these problems. Findings from large scale epidemiological studies have shown that these two conditions are among the most common mental health problems experienced by youth (Armstrong and Costello, 2002; Kandel et al., 1999). Furthermore, substance abusers are frequently involved in various publicly funded social service settings where social workers are likely to be employed (Aarons, Brown, Hough, Garland, and Wood, 2001). Thus, selecting appropriate measures to assess substance abuse and antisocial behaviors is of particular importance in the field of social work.

Advances in measurement of substance abuse and antisocial behaviors have the potential to inform treatment decisions which, in turn, allow for exploring how client characteristics interact with treatment outcomes. For example, some authors have provided evidence that placing youth with conduct problems in group-based treatments had iatrogenic effects (Dishion, McCord, and Poulin, 1999). Thus, easy to use and reliable measures of behavior problems could be helpful for social workers in practice with adolescent substance abusers. Being able to easily identify various risk factors such as these with reliable and valid measures has the potential to improve treatment decisions and client outcomes.

Social workers are frequently required to use the Diagnostic and Statistical Manual (DSM-IV) (American Psychiatric Association, 1994)

diagnoses to justify eligibility for services and capture third party reimbursement. Although the usefulness of such diagnostic systems has been debated by social work scholars (Kutchins and Kirk, 1997; Wakefield, 2002; Wakefield, Pottick, and Kirk, 2002), a clear need exists for standardized instruments that are compatible with DSM-IV language for the simple reason that social workers work in settings where this diagnostic system is required. Although the DSM-IV may not be the best nosological system with social work clients, this system is the current standard in the field and likely the one used by clinicians.

For adults, the Structured Clinical Interview for DSM-IV (SCID; Spitzer et al., 1992) is a semi-structured diagnostic interview that is widely used by clinicians. For adolescents, Frederick Matzner and his colleagues (1994) subsequently developed a prototype version called the KID-SCID. The Structured Clinical Interview for DSM-IV Childhood Diagnoses (KID-SCID, Version 1.0; Hien et al., 1994) is a semi-structured diagnostic interview modeled after the widely used adult version (SCID). Suggested probe questions exist for each DSM-IV criterion, and the interviewer rates the presence of each criterion using three-point ratings (i.e., not present, subthreshold, present, or threshold). This interview is modular, and users may choose which sections are of most interest to them.

The purpose of this study was to examine the inter-rater reliability and convergent validity of the Disruptive Behavior Disorders module (i.e., Attention Deficit Hyperactivity Disorder (ADHD), Conduct Disorder (CD), and Oppositional Defiant Disorder (ODD) and the Substance Abuse Disorders module (i.e., all substance abuse and dependence sections). No published data on the validity or reliability of this instrument are available, since this instrument is still under development. In a small, unpublished evaluation (n = 15) of the reliability between archived diagnoses and those obtained by a KID-SCID interview, Matzner et al. (1997) reported inter-rater reliabilities, as measured by Cohen's kappa (Cohen, 1960), of 0.84, 0.84, and 0.63 for ADHD, CD, and ODD, respectively. Although the initial clinical data on the reliability of the Structured Clinical Interview for DSM-IV (KID-SCID, Version 1.0) seem promising, data on the reliability or validity of this instrument have yet to be published.

This study contributes to the continued validation of this instrument in two important ways. First, this study replicates the previous reliability study by an independent research team in a largely rural state. Thus, this study examines reliability and validity with a different population of adolescents, which could enhance the generalizability of findings.

Furthermore, this validation and reliability study is being conducted by an independent research team with no vested interest in the development of the instrument. Second, this study appears to be the first examination of the convergent validity of the KID-SCID. Thus, the relationships among the DSM-IV criteria and closely related constructs on other established instruments are also a focus of investigation.

This study has important implications for both social work practice and research. Evidence of inter-rater reliability increases researchers' confidence that different interviewers can consistently generate the same results. In clinical settings, using standardized measures can improve the rigor of program evaluation designs, as well as equip program planners with vital data, which can be used to advocate for client needs. Evidence of convergent validity demonstrates that the instrument measures what it purports to measure. Exploring convergent validity is important for research, because this exercise often establishes patterns of relationships between constructs that are useful in theory testing. In clinical practice, knowledge of convergent validity is useful because a greater understanding of relationships between constructs can both help program administrators to select appropriate outcome variables for program evaluation, and develop theoretically-based interventions that target such constructs. Thus, this study has important implications for the KID-SCID's usefulness in both clinical practice and research.

METHOD

A cross-sectional descriptive survey approach was used to psychometrically test the Disruptive Behavior Disorders and Substance Abuse Disorders modules of the KID-SCID. A battery of eight instruments was administered to 50 adolescents receiving residential treatment for substance abuse and severe behavioral problems. In addition to completing the KID-SCID structured interview, participants also completed paper and pencil instruments in a group setting. This study examined available evidence for inter-rater reliability and convergent validity.

Procedure

The university's Institutional Review Board (IRB) reviewed all project procedures and data were not collected until approval was granted. Then, consecutively admitted adolescents were recruited from one residential substance abuse treatment program specializing in the treatment of adolescent substance abusers with behavioral problems. This facility had a dedicated Conduct Disorder unit. Active consent of the adolescent was obtained by having staff at the facility describe the project at intake and then having a separate orientation session for the teens with this research team to reiterate important aspects of the project in order for each adolescent to make an informed decision. Consent from parents was requested by having the adolescent provide consent documents to their parents or guardians during visiting hours. Overall, 73 potential participants were invited to participate, and 50 (68%) adolescents whose parents had initially approved in writing, agreed to participate. Staff at the residential program tracked reasons for not participating. The reasons given were inability to return parental consent forms (n = 8), lack of interest (n = 5), and having no parental involvement (n = 10). Research participants were given a $20 gift card for their involvement in the project.

Once participants were recruited into the study, they completed both a semi-structured mental health and substance abuse interview and a battery of paper-and-pencil measures. A doctoral student with two years of assessment and treatment experience conducted the interview. A second clinician interviewed 18% of the participants (n = 9) and Cohen's kappa (Cohen, 1960) was computed for each diagnosis to ensure reliability. This statistic measures the level of agreement between two clinicians for categorical variables (i.e., diagnosis) and corrects for chance agreement. The battery of paper-and-pencil tests was administered in groups led by the doctoral student.

Participants. Fifty adolescents aged 14 to 18 (m = 16.2; SD = 1.1) participated in this study. In this sample, 70% were male (n = 35), and 30% were female (n = 15). The sample was 86% (n = 43) Caucasian, 6% (n = 3) Biracial-American Indian and White, 4% (n = 2) Biracial-Mexican and White, 2% (n = 1) Biracial-African-American and White, and 2% (n = 1) Mexican.

Measures

To assess the psychometric properties of the KID-SCID instrument with an adolescent population, a study was conducted to evaluate the convergent validity of the KID-SCID with the constructs from the battery of measures used in this study. Other instruments expected to converge with constructs on the KID-SCID were selected based on previous research by our team on comorbid behavior problems and substance abuse. The instruments were 2 diagnostic modules of the KID-

SCID as well as other measures of drug use, i.e., Personal Experience Inventory (PEI) and Problem Oriented Screening Instrument for Teens (POSIT), delinquent behavior (i.e., Self Report Delinquency scales), and mental health problems (i.e., PEI and POSIT).

KID-SCID. Both the Disruptive Behavior Disorders and Substance Abuse Disorders modules of the KID-SCID were used in this study. Although the KID-SCID is consistent with the DSM-IV's categorical approach to diagnosis, a more continuous approach that allows for obtaining convergent validity estimates was employed in this study. Each set of criteria ratings for each symptom was added and then correlated with other continuously scored measures to obtain convergent validity estimates. Each criterion was rated on a 1 to 3 scale ranging from *not present* to *present or threshold.*

Oppositional Defiant Disorder. Eight DSM-IV criteria exist for the diagnosis of Oppositional Defiant Disorder, yielding a scale that ranges from 8 to 24, with higher scores indicating the presence of more criteria. Sample items include *often loses temper* and *often argues with adults.* In this study Cronbach's alpha was 0.63 for this scale. Based on past literature (Martin et al., 1994), it was hypothesized that oppositional defiant criteria would have a positive correlation with the number of conduct disorder criteria, with the Problem Oriented Screening Inventory for Teens' (POSIT) (Radhert, 1991) Mental Health and Aggressive Behavior/Delinquency subscales, and with all scales of delinquent behaving as measured by the Self Report Delinquency Scale (SRD) (Elliott and Ageton, 1980).

Attention Deficit Hyperactivity Disorder. Two sets of criteria clusters exist for Attention Deficit Hyperactivity Disorder (ADHD), and the DSM-IV allows a clinician to specify a subtype of either Primarily Inattentive and/or Primarily Hyperactive. Separate continuous scores were obtained for both the dimensions of inattentiveness and hyperactivity for the purposes of demonstrating convergent validity. Nine criteria exist for the *inattentiveness* dimension of ADHD. The symptom ratings for each criterion (ranging from 1 to 3) were summed to obtain a scale that ranges from 9 to 27, with higher scores indicating the presence of more criteria. Sample items include *often loses things* and *is easily distracted by extraneous stimuli.* In this study, Cronbach's alpha was 0.68 for the inattentiveness criteria. Inattentiveness criteria are hypothesized to correlate positively with hyperactivity criteria, the educational status and mental health subscales on the POSIT, and with the Psychological Disturbance scale of the Personal Experience Inventory (PEI) (Winters and Henly, 1989). Nine criteria also exist for the *hyperactivity* dimension of ADHD. The symptom ratings for each criterion (ranging from 1 to 3) were summed to obtain a scale that ranges from 9 to 27, with higher scores indicating the presence of more criteria. Sample items include *often fidgets* and *acts as if they are always on the go or driven by a motor.* Internal consistency, as measured by Cronbach's alpha, was 0.72 for this scale. Hyperactivity criteria are expected to correlate positively with inattentiveness criteria; with conduct disorder criteria; with indices of delinquency on the SRD; with the mental health, aggressive behavior/ delinquency, and educational status subscales on the POSIT; and with the Psychological Disturbance and Deviant Behavior scales on the PEI.

Conduct Disorder. The DSM-IV lists 15 criteria for the diagnosis of conduct disorder. The symptom ratings were summed to obtain a scale that ranges from 15 to 45, with higher scores indicating the presence of more criteria. Sample items on the conduct disorder scale include *has been physically cruel to people, has been physically cruel to animals,* and *often truant (beginning before age 13).* Internal consistency for this scale was 0.76 in the current study. The conduct disorder criteria are expected to converge with indices of delinquent behavior on the SRD, with the POSIT mental health and aggressive behavior/delinquency subscales, and with the PEI's Uncontrolled and Deviant Behavior scales.

Substance-Related Disorders. In all, the KID-SCID can distinguish among multiple substance-related diagnoses used in clinical practice. For each substance, both Substance Abuse diagnoses and Substance Dependence diagnoses exist. Substance abuse is defined in the DSM-IV (APA, 1994) by four criteria such as *recurrent substance use resulting in failure to fulfill major role obligations at work, school or home,* and *recurrent substance-related legal problems.* Substance Dependence is thought to be a more serious pattern of substance abuse consisting of seven criteria including: *tolerance, withdrawal,* and *taking the substance in larger amounts or over a longer period than was intended.* Substances that are included on the KID-SCID are: Alcohol ($\alpha = 0.84$, dependence; $\alpha = 0.77$, abuse), Marijuana ($\alpha = 0.48$, dependence; $\alpha = 0.24$, abuse), Sedatives ($\alpha = 0.89$, dependence; $\alpha = 0.17$, abuse), Hallucinogens ($\alpha = 0.27$, dependence; $\alpha = 0.07$, abuse), Stimulants ($\alpha = 0.56$, dependence; $\alpha = 0.62$, abuse), Opioids ($\alpha = 0.84$, dependence; $\alpha = 0.13$, abuse), Cocaine ($\alpha = 0.92$, dependence; $\alpha = 0.54$, abuse), Poly-Dependence ($\alpha = 0.45$, dependence; $\alpha = 0.45$, abuse), and Other ($\alpha = 0.84$, dependence; $\alpha = 0.75$, abuse). On the KID-SCID, all criteria are asked for each substance class that the client reports using more than ten times in a single month. The criteria are the same for each substance class despite the fact that some criteria may not apply to certain classes of drugs. For example, the long-held belief that heavy marijuana use has no discernable withdrawal syndrome is only recently being challenged (Kouri and Pope, 2000; Kouri, Pope, and Lukas, 1999). Symptom ratings were summed to obtain scores that ranged from 4 to 12 for substance abuse, and 7 to 21 for substance dependence. Higher scores indicate the presence of more criteria. Both abuse and dependence criteria counts were expected to correlate positively with the POSIT's Substance Use/Abuse subscale and with the PEI's lifetime frequency of use items (i.e., Lifetime, 12-month, and 3-month), the Personal Involvement with Chemicals scale, and Personal Consequences of Use scale.

Self Report Delinquency Scale. The Self Report Delinquency Scale (SRD) (Elliott and Ageton, 1980) is a 47-item instrument in which the respondent indicates the number of times he or she has engaged in a delinquent act. It was developed by rationally selecting categories of juvenile crimes from the Uniform Crime Report. Then, the responses from this self-report instrument were compared to official delinquency statistics in a large sample of juveniles (n = 1,726) involved in the National Youth Survey, a longitudinal study of delinquency. An abbreviated version of the SRD was used in the present study, omitting the seven items pertaining to substance use because of duplication. Examples of offenses included in this measure are *knowingly bought, sold, or held stolen goods (or tried to do any of these things),* and *hit (or threatened to hit) one of your parents.* In past studies, all three delinquency subscales have shown convergent validity with measures of involvement with delinquent peers and conventional bonding (i.e., involvement with family, school, and community) (Elliott, Huizinga, and Ageton, 1985). Furthermore, Elliott and Ageton (1980) reported that the SRD had good internal consistency ($\alpha = 0.91$).

The three subscales used in this study include minor delinquency, index offenses, and general delinquency subscales. Index offenses include nine items about serious aggressive offenses such as *attacked someone with the idea of seriously hurting or killing him or her*, and *had or tried to have sex with someone against their will.* The general delinquency scale contains 24 items covering a wide range of delinquent acts that are less severe than index offenses, but that are thought to be more severe than petty offenses. Sample items include: *Stolen (or tried to steal) a motor vehicle, such as a car or motorcycle, Stolen (or tried to* *steal) something worth more than $50*, and *Sold hard drugs such as heroin, cocaine, or LSD*. The minor delinquency scale is a seven-item scale with items such as *Stolen (or tried to steal) things worth less than five dollars*, and *Been loud, rowdy, or unruly in a public place (disorderly conduct)*.

Personal Experience Inventory. The Personal Experience Inventory (PEI) (Winters and Henly, 1989) is a reliable and valid 276-item inventory measuring drug involvement, psychiatric problems and psychosocial functioning (Winters et al., 1991, 1996, 1999). The scales used in this study include Personal Involvement with Chemicals (29 items) (i.e., frequent use, preoccupation with use, using in inappropriate situations), Personal Consequences (11 items) (i.e., problems with friends, family, or institutions due to use), Uncontrolled (12 items) (i.e., acting out, displaying anger, defying authority), and Deviant Behavior (10 items) (i.e., unlawful and delinquent behavior, acting out at home). In addition to these items, there exists a Frequency of Use item (i.e., Lifetime, 12-month, 3-month) for most classes of substances that asks the participant to rate drug use frequency on a seven point scale ranging from *never* to *40 or more times*.

POSIT. The Problem Oriented Screening Inventory for Teenagers (POSIT) is a reliable and valid screening instrument that is useful in identifying high-risk adolescents in a number of social service settings (Rahdert, 1991). Initial validation (n = 849) by the author showed that for all subscales, higher percentages of adolescents in treatment for substance abuse met clinical cutoffs versus high-school and junior high-school controls (Rahdert, 1991). Hall, Richardson, Spears, and Rembert (1998) showed that the POSIT successfully discriminated between groups of abstaining adolescents and those currently in drug and alcohol treatment.

In this investigation, four subscales from the POSIT were used: the Mental Health scale (22 items), the Educational Status scale (19 items), the Aggressive Behavior/Delinquency scale (16 items), and the Substance Use/Abuse scale (17 items). All items in the POSIT are *yes/no* format, and after raw scores are recoded according to scoring criteria, positive answers within each domain are coded as ones and then summed to yield a total score for each subscale. Ranges thus vary from zero to the number of items included on that subscale, with higher scores indicating more risk in that domain.

Data Analysis

All data were analyzed using SPSS 11.0 (SPSS, 2003). Cohen's Kappa statistic was computed between two independent interviewers completing the KID-SCID diagnostic interviews. Pearson's correlations were computed between the symptom counts of the diagnoses on the KID-SCID and related constructs on the PEI, POSIT, and SRD. All scales were scored using scoring instructions from either the instrument source articles or administration manuals.

Missing data were minimized by reviewing the questionnaires for missing data prior to participants' leaving. Thus, missing data were rare in this study (i.e., less than 3% for any single item on the PEI, POSIT, or SRD and none on the KID-SCID), and missing values were imputed by replacing them with the mean of all other participant responses. Using this procedure was expected to have a minimal impact on the overall findings of this study. Despite using these procedures, one participant did not return a SRD.

RESULTS

Overall Results

Table 1 displays the means and standard deviations for each of the four major instruments used in this study (KID-SCID, POSIT, SRD, and PEI). For each major instrument, the subscales also are listed and the means and standard deviations are identified.

Inter-Rater Reliability

Table 2 presents Cohen's kappa statistic for percentage of agreement between independent raters for all diagnoses. In some cases it was impossible to compute kappa due to no variance in one rater's diagnoses. Under these circumstances the number of agreed upon diagnoses was divided by the total number of diagnoses to obtain a percentage of agreement.

Overall, inter-rater reliability was good for diagnoses in the Disruptive Behavior Disorders and Substance Abuse Disorders modules of the KID-SCID. Kappas were high for both ADHD and ODD, and the percentage of agreement for CD was 100%. For the Substance Abuse Disorders diagnoses, kappas, and percentages of agreement were mostly high, with the exception being those diagnoses with low base rates in the sample (i.e., Opioid Dependence, Sedative Abuse). Thus, higher percentages of agreement and kappas were found for drug classes that were more prevalent in the sample (i.e., marijuana, alcohol, stimulants).

TABLE 1. Client Characteristics by Instrument and Construct: Means and (Standard Deviations)

Construct	Mean (SD)	N
KID-SCID		
Hyperactivity Criteria	14.6 (4.4)	50
Inattentiveness Criteria	15.0 (4.4)	49
ODD Criteria	14.7 (4.0)	49
CD Criteria	26.3 (6.2)	50
Alcohol Dependence	11.1 (4.4)	50
Alcohol Abuse	6.8 (2.9)	50
Cannabis Dependence	16.2 (2.9)	50
Cannabis Abuse	10.4 (1.7)	50
Hallucinogen Dependence	11.9 (2.6)	15*
Hallucinogen Abuse	6.1 (1.6)	15
Cocaine Dependence	13.9 (5.7)	14
Cocaine Abuse	7.7 (2.6)	15
Stimulant Dependence	15.3 (3.3)	24
Stimulant Abuse	8.8 (2.6)	24
Opioid Dependence	11.0 (4.4)	11
Opioid Abuse	5.4 (1.6)	9
Sedative Dependence	10.6 (4.8)	7
Sedative Abuse	5.3 (1.5)	7
Poly-Dependence	17.0 (3.1)	6
Poly-Abuse	10.0 (2.8)	5
Other Dependence	12.6 (4.8)	15
Other Abuse	6.6 (2.7)	15
POSIT		
Mental Health	12.8 (4.9)	50
Substance Abuse	12.2 (3.5)	50
Aggressive/Delinquency	10.2 (3.3)	50
Educational Status	13.6 (4.7)	50
SRD		
Index Offenses	24.9 (49.4)	49
Minor Delinquency	28.2 (34.3)	49
General Delinquency	199.2 (313.1)	49
PEI		
Psychological Disturbance	56.5 (10.1)	50
Deviant Behavior	61.1 (9.4)	50
Personal Involvement	99.8 (10.5)	50
Personal Consequences	26.1 (5.8)	50
Uncontrolled	54.2 (9.0)	50

*N varies for drug dependence and abuse criteria, because prior to enquiring about dependence and abuse criteria a screening is conducted to focus only on substances that a client has reported using.

TABLE 2. Inter-Rater Reliability: Kappa or Percent Agreement for All Diagnoses

Diagnosis	Kappa	% Agreement
ADHD	1.0	--
ODD	.73	--
CD	NA*	100%
Alcohol Dependence	0.77	--
Sedative Dependence	NA	100%
Cannabis Dependence	NA	88%
Stimulant Dependence	NA	100%
Opioid Dependence	0.50	--
Cocaine Dependence	NA	100%
Hallucinogen Dependence	0.40	--
Other Dependence	0.40	--
Alcohol Abuse	1.00	--
Sedative Abuse	NA	50%
Cannabis Abuse	NA	100%
Stimulant Abuse	1.00	--
Opioid Abuse	1.00	--
Cocaine Abuse	NA	100%
Hallucinogen Abuse	NA	66%
Other Abuse	0.40	--

*The kappa statistic cannot be computed when there is no variation in one of the interviewers' diagnoses.

Convergent Validity

Disruptive Behavior Disorders. Overall, the hypothesized pattern of associations between the scales on the Disruptive Behavior Disorders module of the KID-SCID and related constructs was observed. All four scales on this module (i.e., inattentiveness, hyperactivity, oppositional defiant disorder, and conduct disorder) were moderately associated with each other, which has been found in multiple studies on psychiatric comorbidity with adolescents (Costello et al., 1999; Fehon et al., 1997). Each of these scales was also moderately associated with the Mental Health subscale on the POSIT, which was expected since this scale was developed with breadth in mind. That is, it is a screener that covers a range of mental health problems, and should not correlate highly with more specific mental health measures. Finally, all four scales for Disruptive Behavior Disorders was also moderately associated with uncontrolled behavior. Increases in interviewer-rated inattentiveness criteria were associated with increases in reported educational problems on the POSIT and, somewhat surprisingly, associated with increased reports of general delinquency. Increases in the hyperactivity criteria were associated with increased reports of aggressive and delinquent behavior on the POSIT. Participants rated higher on oppositional criteria reported increases in aggressive and delinquent behavior, educational problems, and general delinquency. Finally, higher criteria ratings on the conduct disorder scale were associated with increased reports of index offenses (i.e., serious aggressive crimes), aggressive behavior and delinquency, educational problems, minor delinquency, and deviant behaviors. Table 3 shows the pattern of correlations between the Disruptive Behavior Disorders module of the KID-SCID and select constructs from other measures.

Substance Abuse Disorders. Contrary to the predictions of this study, few significant associations were observed between the number of substance dependence and abuse criteria and the participants' frequency of use. Higher interviewer ratings of criteria for alcohol abuse and dependence, opioid dependence, cocaine dependence and abuse, and hallucinogen abuse were associated with higher self-reported frequency of use. One notable pattern exists for both cannabis abuse and dependence ratings. Near zero magnitude associations emerged between the number of criteria and reported frequency of use. Besides the associations for the cannabis criteria, most correlations, while non-significant, were in the moderate range and in the expected direction. Table 4 shows the associations between the number of interviewer-rated substance abuse and dependence criteria and select measures from the PEI and the POSIT.

Only the number of poly-substance dependence criteria and other substance abuse criteria was associated positively with the Personal Involvement with Chemicals scale from the PEI. These correlations were moderately high to high. These correlations were expected, because the personal involvement scale measures how widespread and varied (i.e., different situations, multiple substances, frequency) one's use is. Thus, it is logical that adolescents reporting use of multiple substances or rare substances on the KID-SCID were found to have high personal involvement with chemicals. Although not statistically significant, most associations were in the low to moderate range and in the expected direction.

Three statistically significant, positive associations emerged between dependence and abuse criteria and the Personal Consequences of Use scale on the PEI. These included stimulant dependence ($r = 0.37$, $p < .01$), cannabis abuse ($r = 0.32$, $p < .01$), and other abuse ($r = 0.64$, $p <$

TABLE 3. Convergent Validity of Disruptive Behavior Disorders Criteria: Correlation Coefficients

	Hyperactivity	Inattentiveness	Oppositional	Conduct
POSIT				
Mental Health	.44**	.53**	.48**	.44**
Aggressive/Del.	.30*	.18	.45**	.63**
Education	.20	.62**	.39**	.33*
SRD				
Index Offenses	.08	.15	.25	.51**
Minor	.18	.24	.25	.39**
General	.04	.46**	.33*	.14
PEI				
Psychological Disturbance	.27	.36*	.22	.31*
Deviant Behavior	.23	.08	.20	.58**
Uncontrolled	.39**	.42**	.50**	.51**
KID-SCID				
Hyperactivity	-			
Inattentiveness	.46**	-		
ODD	.56**	.50**	-	
CD	.30*	.24	.45**	-

**Correlation is significant at the 0.01 level (2-tailed).
*Correlation is significant at the 0.05 level (2-tailed).
Note: all figures presented are Pearson's bivariate correlations.

.01). Most other associations, while non-significant, were moderately related with Personal Consequences of Use and in the hypothesized direction.

Six statistically significant, positive associations existed between the POSIT Substance Abuse/Use subscale and the dependence and abuse criteria ratings of the KID-SCID. In all cases, higher interviewer-rated number of criteria on the KID-SCID was associated with increased self report of more alcohol and drug-related risk factors on the POSIT. Significant associations were observed for alcohol dependence ($r = 0.33$, $p < .05$), alcohol abuse ($r = 0.38$, $p < .01$), cannabis dependence ($r = 0.42$, $p < .01$), cannabis abuse ($r = 0.31$, $p < .05$), stimulant dependence ($r = 0.35$, $p < .05$), and other abuse ($r = 0.53$, $p < .05$).

TABLE 4. Convergent Validity of Substance-Related Disorders of the KID-SCID

	Lifetime Frequency (PEI)	12-month Frequency (PEI)	3-month Frequency (PEI)	Personal Involvement (PEI)	Personal Consequences (PEI)	Substance Abuse (POSIT)
Dependence						
Alcohol	.46**	.46**	.23	.24	.23	.33*
Cannabis	−.06	.11	−.09	.21	.21	.42**
Hallucinogen	.23	.34	.29	.51	.47	.49
Cocaine	.62*	.74*	.44	.30	.30	.12
Stimulant	.24	.29	.29	.19	.37**	.35*
Opioid	.79**	.79**	.79**	.50	.65	.60
Sedative	NA***	NA	NA	.06	.67	.46
Other	NA	NA	NA	.50	.40	.33
Poly	NA	NA	NA	.95**	.53	.30
Abuse						
Alcohol	.46**	.42**	.35*	.24	.17	.38**
Cannabis	.05	.03	.00	.16	.32*	.31*
Hallucinogen	.56*	.77**	.44	.23	.37	.27
Cocaine	.50	.89**	.60*	.16	.26	.18
Stimulant	.33	.29	.30	.13	.33	.22
Opioid	.58	.56	.56	.55	.63	.55
Sedative	NA	NA	NA	.23	.65	.44
Other	NA	NA	NA	.64*	.64**	.53*
Poly	NA	NA	NA	.77	.63	.37

***No matching Frequency of Use Question available on the PEI.
**Correlation is significant at the 0.01 level (2-tailed).
*Correlation is significant at the 0.05 level (2-tailed).
Note: all figures presented are Pearson's bivariate correlations.

DISCUSSION

For the three most commonly used substances in this sample (i.e., alcohol, cannabis, and stimulants) inter-rater reliability was high. For example, kappas of 0.77, 1.0, and 1.0 were found for Alcohol Dependence, Alcohol Abuse, and Stimulant Abuse, respectively. Percentages of agreement were 88%, 100%, and 100% for Cannabis Dependence, Cannabis Abuse, and Stimulant Dependence, respectively. Because of the small number of cases that "passed" the screener and were assessed for other substance-related diagnoses, some of the other estimates of inter-rater reliability may appear deceptively low. Nevertheless, this study found high inter-rater reliability for substances that epidemiological studies have found to be most commonly used among adolescents (Johnston, O'Malley, and Bachman, 2003), which seems to be an important finding that overshadows lower estimates of inter-rater reliability found for the criteria of the lesser used classes of drugs. These latter estimates would be very sensitive to any disagreement, and should be viewed cautiously.

The convergent validity analyses of the Disruptive Behavior Disorders module of the KID-SCID produced results largely as expected. Higher ratings of KID-SCID criteria for ODD, ADHD, and CD were associated with more reported mental health problems on the POSIT as well as more uncontrolled behaviors as measured by the PEI. Inattentiveness was correlated moderately high ($r = 0.62$, $p < .01$) with educational status, which is consistent with past work on this symptom cluster. Surprisingly, higher ratings of inattentiveness were related to higher reports of general delinquency as well. One possible explanation for this comes from models which suggest that early school failure predicts later delinquency (Hawkins, Catalano, and Miller, 1992). Previous studies have shown that hyperactivity and conduct problems may have similar etiological roots (Patterson, DeGarmo, and Knutson, 2000), but less work linking inattentiveness with conduct problems exists. This could also be an artifact of measurement, which would disappear if partial correlations controlling for the presence of hyperactivity were done. Because the scope of this article was initial instrument validation, these types of analyses were not done. Other findings of note in this analysis include that higher ratings of conduct disorder criteria were associated with self-reported problems on all scales except for general delinquency. This finding is consistent with the portrait painted by the empirical literature regarding the severe behavioral problems associated with CD. Also, it is notable that children with higher ratings of ODD criteria reported higher general delinquency, but a higher number of ODD criteria was not significantly associated with serious aggressive crimes as measured by the index offences scale. This finding is consistent with the literature showing that conduct disorder and ODD are discrete constructs, and that ODD is associated with younger children which possibly progresses into CD and a more severe behavioral profile at later ages (Quay, 1999). In summary, good support for convergent validity of the Disruptive Behavior Disorders scales of the KID-SCID was found that also is consistent with major themes in the literature.

Several explanations are possible for the pattern of associations observed between substance abuse and dependence criteria and frequency of use, personal consequences of use and the POSIT subscale that measures global substance abuse problems. First, the absence of an association could be a result of low power due to the low base rates for many classes of substances. This notion is supported by two patterns in the data. Higher interviewer-rated criteria for the three most commonly used substances (i.e., marijuana, alcohol, and stimulants) were associated with higher ratings of global problems with substance use and abuse as measured by the POSIT. Also, many of the criteria ratings for the other substances were in the expected direction and sometimes close to significant when alpha was set at the 0.05 level. Thus, it could be that the small sample size resulted in some spurious correlations as well as some true correlations that failed to reach significance. This explanation cannot, however, account for the lack of associations between cannabis dependence and abuse criteria ratings and self-reported ratings of frequency of use, because every participant (n = 50) met the screening criteria on the KID-SCID for marijuana and was asked the abuse and dependence questions for this substance. The finding that cannabis dependence and abuse symptoms were not correlated with frequency of use could also be due to adolescents simply not attributing their problems to this drug in favor of "harder" drugs that they reported using. Thus, this finding could speak to adolescents' perceived risk of using marijuana. It could also be possible, but counterintuitive, that sometimes using a lot of one substance does not result in dependence or abuse as defined by the DSM-IV. Finally, the possibility exists that a range restriction limits the magnitude of correlations. The inpatient population in this study was severe on many problem dimensions, and there may not have been enough variation to detect some correlations, as opposed to a scenario in which a wider variety of substance abusing adolescents was interviewed. In summary, although a sporadic pattern of correlations was observed between number of dependence and abuse criteria and frequency of use, Personal Involvement with Chemicals, and Personal Consequences of Use, significant positive correlations existed between the three most commonly used drugs and global substance abuse problems as measured by the POSIT.

CONCLUSIONS

This study marks an important step in establishing the validity and reliability of the Disruptive Behavior Disorders and Substance Abuse

Disorders modules of the KID-SCID. In summary, good evidence for convergent validity and inter-rater reliability was found for the Disruptive Behavior Disorders module and the more common substance classes in the Substance Abuse Disorders module of the KID-SCID.

Although these data are supportive of the use of the KID-SCID, the study is limited in several ways. First, because of the small sample size it is possible that spurious correlations exist between some of the more uncommonly used drugs and the other major constructs tested in this article. Second, the KID-SCID was administered to a racially homogenous group of adolescents with severe behavioral and substance abuse problems, which then limits the generalizability of these findings. Future validation work with this instrument should include samples of adolescents diverse on both demographic and clinical characteristics. Also, this work only investigated two facets of the overall reliability and validity of this measure. To truly be useful in clinical practice, a measure should allow clinicians to generate empirically supported inferences, which can usually only be achieved by a lengthy process of data collection and testing (Springer, Abell, and Hudson, 2002). Future work should focus on using other methods of establishing the validity, reliability, and utility of the KID-SCID, such as the known groups approach, factorial analysis, and sensitivity and specificity analyses. Finally, because of the large number of correlations conducted, it is possible that some Type I errors were committed due to familywise error rates (Hays, 1994). To address this issue, we used Hays' (1994) formula for maximum familywise error (see Equations 1 and 2). By using this formula we obtained an adjusted alpha of .021 for the Disruptive Behavior Disorders correlations (α planned comparison = .05; K = 42) and an adjusted alpha of .01 for the substance use frequency correlations (α planned comparison = .05; K = 90).

$$\alpha_{FW} = 1 - (1 - \alpha_{PC})^K \qquad (1)$$
$$\alpha_{PC} = \alpha_{FW}/K \qquad (2)$$

Using these conservative adjustments would not change the main findings regarding the convergent validity of the disruptive behavior disorders module, as 20 of 25 correlations would remain significant were alpha adjusted to .021. It is more difficult to interpret the pattern among the substance use frequency correlations due to the large number of tests conducted (i.e., 90). Nevertheless, the overall impact of using this alpha level would be most pronounced on the low base rate substances due to the lack of overall power. One further limitation of this study was the possible impact of our procedure for obtaining parental consent. Of the 23 clients who were invited to participate but did not eventually participate, 78% were due to a lack of parental involvement or inability to obtain parental consent. Past studies on family relationships in early adolescence have shown that requiring parental consent can systematically exclude higher severity families (Weinberger, Tublin, Ford, and Feldman, 1990). It is uncertain how active parental consenting procedures impacted these data. Finally, it is possible that administering instruments to a group of adolescents could have produced cohort effects. Efforts to prevent this included close proctoring of groups that limited discussion between participants, and documenting questions asked about items, so that consistent administration was maintained across groups.

In conclusion, this study has provided initial data on the inter-rater reliability and convergent validity of select modules of the KID-SCID. Despite the need for greater refinement and testing, the evidence supports the use of the Disruptive Behavior Disorders and Substance Abuse Disorders modules of the KID-SCID in social work practice with adolescents. Future work on the validation of this instrument with larger and more diverse samples is highly desirable. Future work on the relationship between frequency of use and diagnostic criteria for substance abuse and dependence is also warranted based on the findings of this study.

REFERENCES

Aarons, G. A., Brown, S. A., Hough, R. L., Garland, A. F., & Wood, P. A. (2001). Prevalence of adolescent substance use disorders across five sectors of care. *Journal of the American Academy of Child & Adolescent Psychiatry, 40*(4), 419-426.

American Psychiatric Association (1994). *Diagnostic and statistical manual of mental disorders (4th edition).* Washington, DC: Author.

Armstrong, T. D., & Costello, E. (2002). Community studies on adolescent substance use, abuse, or dependence and psychiatric comorbidity. *Journal of Consulting & Clinical Psychology, 70*(6), 1224-1239.

Cohen, J. (1960). A coefficient of agreement for nominal scales. *Educational & Psychological Measurement, 20,* 37-46.

Costello, E., Erkanli, A., Federman, E., & Angold, A. (1999). Development of psychiatric comorbidity with substance abuse in adolescents: Effects of timing and sex. *Journal of Clinical Child Psychology, 28*(3), 298-311.

Dishion, T., McCord, J., & Poulin, F. (1999). When interventions harm: Peer groups and problem behavior. *American Psychologist, 54*(9), 755-764.

Elliott, D. S., & Ageton, S. S. (1980). Reconciling race and class differences in self-reported and official estimates of delinquency. *American Sociological Review, 45,* 95-110.

Elliott, D. S., Huizinga, D., & Ageton, S. S. (1985). *Explaining delinquency and drug abuse.* Beverly Hills: Sage Publications.

Fehon, D. C., Becker, D. F., Grilo, C. M., & Walker, M. L. (1997). Diagnostic comorbidity in hospitalized adolescents with conduct disorder. *Comprehensive Psychiatry, 38*(3), 141-145.

Hall, J. A., Richardson, B., Spears, J., & Rembert, J. K. (1998). Validation of the POSIT: Comparing drug using and abstaining youth. *Journal of Child & Adolescent Substance Abuse, 8*(2), 29-61.

Hawkins, J. D., Catalano, R. F., & Miller, J. (1992). Risk and protective factors for alcohol and other drug problems in adolescence and early adulthood: Implications for substance abuse prevention. *Psychological Bulletin, 112,* 64-105.

Hays, W. L. (1994). *Statistics (Fifth edition).* Fort Worth, TX: Harcourt Brace College Publishers.

Hien, D., Matzner, F. J., First, M. B., Spitzer, R. L., Williams, J., & Gibbon, M. (1994). *Structured Clinical Interview for DSM-IV Childhood Diagnoses (KID-SCID).* New York, Biometrics Research presentation.

Johnston, L. D., O'Malley, P. M., & Bachman, J. G. (2003). *Monitoring the future national survey results on drug use, 1975-2002. Volume I: Secondary school students (NIH Publication No. 03-5375).* Bethesda, MD: National Institute on Drug Abuse.

Kandel, D. B., Johnson, J. G., Bird, H. R., Weissman, M. M., Goodman, S. H., Lahey, B. B. et al. (1999). Psychiatric comorbidity among adolescents with substance use disorders: Findings from the MECA study. *Journal of the American Academy of Child & Adolescent Psychiatry, 38*(6), 693-699.

Kouri, E. M., & Pope, H. G. (2000). Abstinence symptoms during withdrawal from chronic marijuana use. *Experimental & Clinical Psychopharmacology, 8*(4), 483-492.

Kouri, E. M., Pope, H. G., & Lukas, S. E. (1999). Changes in aggressive behavior during withdrawal from long-term marijuana use. *Psychopharmacology, 143*(3), 302-308.

Kutchins, H., & Kirk, S. A. (1997). *Making us crazy: DSM: The psychiatric bible and the creation of mental disorders.* New York: Free Press.

Martin, C. S., Earleywine, M., Blackson, T. C., Vanyukov, M. M. et al. (1994). Aggressivity, inattention, hyperactivity, and impulsivity in boys at high and low risk for substance abuse. *Journal of Abnormal Child Psychology, 22*(2), 177-203.

Matzner, F. J., Silva, R., Silvan, M., Chowdhury, M., & Nastasi, L. (1997). *Preliminary test-retest reliability of the KID-SCID.* Paper presented at the Scientific Proceedings of the American Academy of Child and Adolescent Psychiatry.

Patterson, G. R., DeGarmo, D. S., & Knutson, N. (2000). Hyperactive and antisocial behaviors: Comorbid or two points in the same process? *Development & Psychopathology, 12*(1), 91-106.

Quay, H. C. (1999). Classification of the disruptive behavior disorders. In H. C. Quay & A. E. Hogan (Eds.), *Handbook of disruptive behavior disorders* (pp. 3-21). New York: Kluwer Academic/Plenum Publishers.

Rahdert, E. (1991). *Adolescent assessment & referral system*. Washington, DC: National Institute on Drug Abuse.

Reebye, P., Moretti, M. M., & Lessard, J. C. (1995). Conduct disorder and substance use disorder: Comorbidity in a clinical sample of preadolescents and adolescents. *Canadian Journal of Psychiatry, 40*(6), 313-319.

Spitzer, R. L., Williams, J. B., Gibbon, M., & First, M. B. (1992). The Structured Clinical Interview for DSM-III-R (SCID): I. History, rationale, and description. *Archives of General Psychiatry, 49*(8), 624-629.

Springer, D. W., Abell, N., & Hudson, W. W. (2002). Creating and validating rapid assessment instruments for practice and research: Part 1. *Research on Social Work Practice,* 12(3), 408-439.

SPSS. (2003). *SPSS Version 11.0*. Chicago, IL: Author.

Wakefield, J. C. (2002). Values and the validity of diagnostic criteria: Disvalued versus disordered conditions of childhood and adolescence. In J. Z. Sadler (Ed.), *Descriptions and prescriptions: Values, mental disorders, and the DSMs* (pp. 148-164). Baltimore, MD: Johns Hopkins University Press.

Wakefield, J. C., Pottick, K. J., & Kirk, S. A. (2002). Should the DSM-IV diagnostic criteria for conduct disorder consider social context? *American Journal of Psychiatry, 159*(3), 380-386.

Weinberger, D. A., Tublin, S. K., Ford, M. E., & Feldman, S. S. (1990). Preadolescents' social-emotional adjustment and selective attrition in family research. *Child Development, 61,* 1374-1386.

Winters, K. C., & Henly, G. A. (1989). *Personal experience inventory–A measure of substance abuse in adolescents*. Los Angeles, CA: Western Psychological Services.

Winters, K. C., Latimer, W. W., Stinchfield, R. D., & Henly, G. (1999). Assessing adolescent drug use with the Personal Experience Inventory. In M. E. Maruish (Ed.), *The use of psychological testing for treatment planning and outcomes assessment (2nd ed.)* (pp. 599-630). Mahwah, NJ: Lawrence Erlbaum Associates.

Winters, K. C., Stinchfield, R., & Henly, G. A. (1996). Convergent and predictive validity of scales measuring adolescent substance abuse. *Journal of Child & Adolescent Substance Abuse, 5*(3), 37-55.

Winters, K. C., Stinchfield, R. D., Henly, G. A., & Schwartz, R. H. (1991). Validity of adolescent self-report of alcohol and drug involvement. *The International Journal of the Addictions,* 25(11A), 1379-1395.

Using Self-Rating Scales for Assessing the Severely Mentally Ill Client: A Clinical and Psychometric Perspective

Edward H. Taylor

SUMMARY. Seventy-five SPMI clients were administered Hudson's *Generalized Contentment Scale* and *Index of Self-Esteem*. The item responses and total scores were analyzed statistically for reliability and validity. It was found that when a guided self-rating system rather than independent self-rating was employed, the two Hudson scales had high reliability (.88 and .91) and concurrent instrument validity (.88 and .91). Limited construct validity was also established. In addition, the article explains how the guided self-ratings are conducted and provides suggestions for managing symptoms during the assessment. *[Article copies available for a fee from The Haworth Document Delivery Service: 1-800-HAWORTH. E-mail address: <docdelivery@haworth press.com> Website: <http://www.HaworthPress.com> © 2005 by The Haworth Press, Inc. All rights reserved.]*

Edward H. Taylor, PhD, LICSW, is affiliated with the School of Social Work, University of Minnesota, Saint Paul, MN.

Address correspondence to: Edward H. Taylor, PhD, LICSW, School of Social Work, Peters Hall, University of Minnesota, Twin Cities Campus, 1404 Gortner Avenue, Saint Paul, MN 55108 (E-mail: ehtaylor@che.umn.edu).

[Haworth co-indexing entry note]: "Using Self-Rating Scales for Assessing the Severely Mentally Ill Client: A Clinical and Psychometric Perspective." Taylor, Edward H. Co-published simultaneously in *Journal of Human Behavior in the Social Environment* (The Haworth Social Work Practice Press, an imprint of The Haworth Press, Inc.) Vol. 11, No. 3/4, 2005, pp. 23-40; and: *Approaches to Measuring Human Behavior in the Social Environment* (ed: William R. Nugent) The Haworth Social Work Practice Press, an imprint of The Haworth Press, Inc., 2005, pp. 23-40. Single or multiple copies of this article are available for a fee from The Haworth Document Delivery Service [1-800-HAWORTH, 9:00 a.m. - 5:00 p.m. (EST). E-mail address: docdelivery@haworthpress.com].

Available online at http://www.haworthpress.com/web/JHBSE
doi:10.1300/J137v11n03_02

KEYWORDS. Generalized Contentment Scale, Index of Self-Esteem, reliability, schizophrenia, severe and persistent mental illness, validity

This study explored the efficacy of using depression and similar self-rating scales with clients who have severe schizophrenia and whether clinical procedures or instructions must be significantly changed before severely mentally ill clients can complete self-rating instruments. A literature review found that none of the depression rating scales most widely used in the past ten years have been studied for reliability and validity with individuals who have schizophrenia and extremely severe chronic symptoms. The ability of individuals with mild versus severe symptoms to report problems may differ greatly. This is particularly true when one considers the amount of abstract thinking required for completing self-rating scales. Clients must determine the question's meaning, contextually relate each item to their personal situation, and quickly transform responses into broad ranking numerical categories. In addition, scales tend to infer rather than explicitly define time and boundaries. Therefore, completing self-rating scales becomes more difficult as a client's thoughts are disrupted by increased anxiety, hallucinations, and delusions. Nonetheless, economically tracking when and how depression symptoms change in people with the most severe forms of schizophrenia is highly advantageous for clinical programs, families, and the individual client. Accurate self-rating scales can assist in evaluating treatment effectiveness and help identify clients who are at an increased risk for suicide.

Suicide is the highest cause of premature deaths for people with schizophrenia (Nicole & Shriqui, 1995). Torrey (2001) states that depression is the best explanation for suicide among people with schizophrenia and that at some point almost all clients with schizophrenia will experience significant feelings of depression.

The combination of depression and schizophrenia can increase a client's cognitive confusion, obsessive thinking, and feelings of hopelessness (Torrey, 2001; Hale & Hale, 1995). In addition, severe schizophrenia also depletes a person's objectivity, concentration, and skills for comprehending instructions. Therefore, clients with the most severe symptoms may require additional instructions and assistance in completing self-rating instruments. Presently it is unknown whether guidance from a social worker changes the scales' reliability and validity. Furthermore, little or no research has been reported on how self-rating scales can be therapeutically presented to clients in this diagnostic category.

Accurately assessing depression in clients with schizophrenia is difficult. By definition, schizophrenia creates symptoms that mimic depressive indicators. Classical signs such as blunted affect, isolation, reduced concentration, restlessness, and sleeping difficulties can be observed in clients with schizophrenia and those with depression. We also know that a person can simultaneously have both disorders (Taylor, 1997). Clinically sound self-rating scales have the potential for screening or assessing severely mentally ill clients' depressive symptoms and economically tracking changes in these symptoms over time and across treatment modalities. Understandably, the employment of self-rating scales can become very tempting for both clinicians and organizations. Self-rating instruments can help organizations inexpensively meet quality assurance and outcome evaluation standards. In addition, community treatment for clients with serious mental disorders is also stimulating interest in self-rating scales. Social workers, as an example, know that clients may avoid psychiatric hospitalizations and receive more intense outpatient treatment if the individual's increasing symptoms are quickly identified, accurately measured, and convincingly documented (Black & Andreasen, 1999). Therefore, case managers and therapists are constantly searching for tools that can distinguish shifts in a client's social functioning, mood, anxiety, or thought processes. As a result, instruments like those found in Hudson's (1982) Clinical Measurement Package are extremely popular among social workers.

The Clinical Measurement Package consists of nine self-rating scales designed to screen for the presence and intensity of mental or social adjustment problems. These instruments were specifically designed to provide social workers with psychometrically sound tools for evaluating community programs and identifying clients who did not have a psychotic disorder but may benefit from a mental health assessment. Hudson's original reliability and validity studies were completed with people who were free of psychoses. Furthermore, the manual advises that the instruments may not maintain their psychometric properties when used for assessing individuals who have psychotic episodes (Hudson, 1982). Nonetheless, clinicians and researchers are incorporating the self-rating scales into their evaluations of clients with severe and persistent mental illness. For example, three of the scales were used in a schizophrenia medication study (Grebb et al., 1986). Furthermore, when visiting clinics this researcher found the Hudson instruments are often used for assessing mentally ill clients who have a history of psychosis. The fact that these instruments are widely distributed, published in several textbooks, easy to score, and taught in seminars increases the probability of their use with clients who have psychotic disorders. Assessment tools that are incorrectly used or lack reliability and validity can give dangerous and misleading information. The use of an inappropriate mood or suicide rating scale, as an example, may tragically fail to reflect the client's immediate potential for self-harm. Therefore, it is paramount for us to learn whether depression instruments like Hudson's Generalized Contentment Scale can be appropriately used for assessing mentally ill clients who have a severe psychosis.

PURPOSE AND SAMPLE

This was an exploratory investigation to determine whether clients who have extremely severe schizophrenia can self-rate their symptoms and whether it is psychometrically appropriate to use Hudson's Generalized Contentment Scale (GCS) with severely and persistently mentally ill (SPMI) clients. This study used the original Hudson instruments containing a 5-point response scale. Because clients with SPMI often have concentration and attention problems, the newer revised Hudson instruments containing a 7-point response scale were not employed. Both editions of the Clinical Measurement Package Scales can be obtained from WALMYR, the current publisher. Seventy-five adults with severe schizophrenia volunteered for this project. The sample is distinguished by the subjects' high severity of illness and diagnostic verification. Because this project recruited individuals who were part of a larger National Institute of Mental Health funded neuroscience research study, it was possible to have a very narrow and specific inclusion policy. This insured the participants had similar symptoms, severity levels, and cognitive skills. However, in order to insure that all participants were voluntary, correctly medicated, and matched for illness severity, the sample could not be randomized. This is an accidental sample in which the participants were certified through interviews, semi-structured assessments, and medical records to meet the following criteria. Each subject was required to have: (1) a diagnosis of schizophrenia confirmed by two or more independent psychiatrists and assessments; (2) chronic schizophrenia for four or more years; (3) almost daily psychotic symptoms; (4) psychotic symptoms that continued while on psychotropic medications; (5) an inability to hold a full or part time job for the past two or more years; and (6) not lived independently or in a supervised apartment for the past two or more years. Therefore, every subject resided with a family or in a group home and was unable to perform structured volunteer work or part-time employment. They were able to participate in day hospitals and in limited psychosocial clubhouse activities and accept medical treatment. In order to take part in this study, the participants were further required to: (1) comply with individualized medication treatment recommendations; (2) have received the same medication and dosage for the past three months; and, (3) currently be experiencing no crisis, new environmental stressors, or treatment changes (includes psychosocial, rehabilitation, and medical service interventions). This set of criteria was imposed to ensure that the research focused on individuals who were experiencing symptoms related primarily to schizophrenia rather than a psychosocial stressor or changes in medications.

The sample consisted of 19 females and 56 males between the ages of 19 and 51 years of age with a mean age of 28.7 (sd = 5.8). Only 2 females and 12 males identified themselves as being a racial or cultural minority, and the entire sample had grown-up as children and adolescents in lower-middle to upper-middle income families. That is, neither the subjects, their families, nor medical records indicated that any of the participants had lived in poverty as a child or prior to the onset of schizophrenia. Only 4 of the individuals had not received a high school diploma, and none had completed a college degree or technical training program. All seventy-five subjects were considered to be partially medication resistant. In other words, neuroleptic drugs decreased, but did not completely do away with the person's positive and negative symptoms. All of the participants had difficulties with hallucinations, delusions, concentration, social judgment, memory, isolation, communications, interpersonal relationships, social perceptions, and social problem-solving. This is the first study to explore whether clients who must actively contend with disruptive psychotic and negative symptoms can reliably complete self-rating scales.

RESEARCH DESIGN

This study addresses the following questions: (1) do self-rating scales maintain their psychometric values when completed by individuals with severe schizophrenia; and (2) are specialized instructions and clinical techniques required for administering self-rating scales to severely mentally ill clients? Each research participant was given Hudson's Generalized Contentment Scale (GCS), Index of Self-Esteem (ISE), Psycho-Social Screening Package (PSSP), as well as the Zung Depression Scale (Zung, 1965) and Rosenberg Self-Esteem Scale (Rosenberg, 1965). The Zung and Rosenberg scales were adopted because they are extremely short (fewer than 25 items each) and, like the Hudson scales, require forced-choice responses. Furthermore, the Zung scale was used in the reliability and validity studies originally reported by Hudson (1982). The study additionally administered the Negative Symptoms Rating Scale (NSRS) to each client. The NSRS (Jaeger, Kirch, & Wyatt, 1986) consists of questions and memory tasks that are verbally presented and scored by the clinician. As a final step, a trained observer using the Psychiatric Symptom Assessment Scale (Bigelow & Berthot, 1989) rated each individual's symptoms several hours prior to or after the GCS and ISE were administered. The Psychiatric Symptom Assessment Scale (PSAS) is a modification of the Brief Psychiatric Rating Scale (Overall & Gorham, 1962) and was developed specifically for measuring schizophrenia or psychotic symptoms. With the exception of the PSAS and intelligence testing, all instruments were administered by the researcher. Wechsler intelligence scores were gained from clinic records after all research measurements had been completed.

Twenty of the 75 participants were initially introduced to the GCS scale and requested to independently complete and return the form within 24 hours. Standardized instructions were given verbally to each person in a private room. None of the instruments were given in a group setting. The instructions and training from the researcher included: (a) reading aloud the GCS's published instructions; (b) answering participant questions about the scale; (c) insuring participants could read and understand the questions; (d) providing examples of how to use the GCS's 1 through 5 response system; and (e) supervising a practice session with an instrument similar to the Hudson Scales. The practice instrument consisted of five questions developed by the researcher. Care was taken to insure the practice items were substantially different from the actual research instruments and free of depression and self-esteem content. However, no assistance or structure for answering the GCS questions was provided. The 20 subjects were encouraged to answer privately all 25 items during the remaining part of the day or that evening. The completed form was to be returned to the researcher the next day. Their case managers were requested to remind each person to complete and return the form but not to assist in answering the questions. When the participant responses were examined, it became clear that self-ratings could not be used without additional assistance and structure. The following errors were noted in the 20 piloted GCS forms: none of the participants completed all 25 items; 4 individuals used numerical answers above the instrument's response range; 11 people answered four or less items; and 3 participants recorded several illegible responses. As a result, a guided self-rating method was developed and used with all 75 participants. The instructions and method used for helping clients complete each self-rating scale are provided in the appendix.

PSYCHOMETRICALLY TESTING
THE GUIDED SELF-RATING METHOD

Reliability was studied using Cronbach's Coefficient Alpha and the test-retest method. Cronbach's Coefficient Alpha is considered one of the better statistical methods for establishing an instrument's internal consistency (Nunnally & Bernstein, 1994; Hudson, 1982). An alpha coefficient represents the mean or average of all possible split-half correlations that can be performed with an instrument. The test-retest method estimates reliability by administering the same scale to clients twice. Scores from the first and second assessments are then correlated. Reliability is commonly defined as the ability for an instrument to accurately replicate identical or similar results over numerous replications. Cronbach's Coefficient Alpha was calculated for the six scales listed in Table 1, and a test-retest reliability estimate was completed for the Generalized Contentment Scale and the Index of Self-Esteem. There was a 14-day delay before the scales were administered again. Throughout this period, the participants continued to have chronic positive and negative symptoms. A two-week waiting period was used to better determine whether the instruments' internal consistency remained intact over an extended period of time. Because the clients have so many severe symptoms, it was important to insure the responses were stable over time. Measurements taken from one day to the next or within the same week may reflect temporary problems or improvements linked to the immediate environment, medications, or other factors, rather than an actual clinical depression.

There are several types of validity that need to be examined before a scale can be trusted for clinical assessments. It is almost impossible for a single study to measure meaningfully all validity forms relating to an instrument. This study was only able to heuristically investigate whether the concurrent instrument validity and construct validity of the Generalized Contentment Scale and Index of Self-Esteem remained acceptable

TABLE 1. Reliability Coefficients (Cronbach's Alpha)

Hudson's General Contentment Scale	.883
Hudson's Index of Self-Esteem	.913
Negative Symptom Rating Scale	.890
Rosenberg Self-Esteem Scale	.897
Zung Depression Scale	.731
Psychiatric Symptom Assessment Scale	.895

when used with severely mentally ill clients. Concurrent instrument validity is a form of criterion validity that tells a social worker if an instrument is predicting a specific quality, criterion or related symptom group such as depression or self-esteem. Psychometrically concurrent instrument validity is established when a scale known to measure an identified criterion (i.e., depression) highly correlates with an experimental scale (Nunnally & Bernstein, 1994; Hudson, 1982). Unfortunately, none of the instruments used for this project have been validated with severely mentally ill subjects. Therefore, we can correlate scores between the Generalized Contentment Scale and Zung Depression Scale, and between the Index of Self-Esteem and Rosenberg Self-Esteem Scale. If the two sets of scales are highly correlated, we will have heuristically, but not psychometrically, established an indication of concurrent instrument validity. That is, we will be a step closer to validating the instrument but cannot be certain we are actually measuring depression and self-esteem in clients who have schizophrenia.

Construct validity helps the clinician determine whether an instrument is sensitive to or measures important factors that are commonly theorized to be part of a psychological or behavioral attribute (Nunnally & Bernstein, 1994; Hudson, 1982). For example, one would anticipate, based on studies of mood disorders, that factors like sadness, unhappiness, and sleeplessness would correlate more highly with depression than age, gender, or intellectual capacity. For this study, Hudson's original 1982 model was followed. Three classes of variables expected to correlate at a high, moderate and low level of association with the Generalized Contentment Scale and Index of Self-Esteem are identified in Table 2. Hudson (1982) suggested that scales with construct validity would correlate poorly (Class III) with social background and demographic type variables; moderately (Class II) with variables that are only partially related to the scale's construct; and highly (Class I) with variables that are intricately related to the construct. Therefore, as shown in Table 2, it was hypothesized the Generalized Contentment Scale (GCS) and Index of Self-Esteem (ISE) would correlate highest among the GCS, ISE, Zung, and Rosenberg total scale scores and a single item rating of depression and self-esteem taken from Hudson's Psycho-Social Screening Package (PSSP). Class II variables consist of PSSP items concerning work, relationships, and identity that relate more generally to depression and self-esteem as well as the total scale scores for the PSSP and Negative Symptoms Scale.

The PSSP requires clients to rate how often they are concerned about depression, unhappiness, work quality, anxiety, and interpersonal relationships. Each PSSP item is rated from 1 (almost never experienced) to 5 (almost always experienced). Scores from two PSSP items asking "I feel depressed" and "I have a low sense of self-esteem" were hypothe-

TABLE 2. Criterion Variables by Expected Class for Estimating GCS & ISE Scales' Construct Validity

	GCS Construct Validity	ISE Construct Validity
Class I (high association expected)		
Hudson's General Contentment Scale	N/A	0.958
Hudson's Index of Self-Esteem	0.958	N/A
Zung Depression Scale	0.907	0.880
Rosenberg Self-Esteem	0.784	0.748
PSAS Observed Depression Rating	0.391	0.419
Depression Self-Rating (Item 1: Hudson's PSSP)	0.681	0.705
Self-Esteem Self-Rating (Item 2: Hudson's PSSP)	0.498	0.518
Class II (moderate association expected)		
Negative Symptoms Scale	0.213	0.239
PSAS Global Score	0.389	0.167
Family Relationships (Item 15: Hudson's PSSP)	0.279	0.446
Work Quality (Item 12: Hudson's PSSP)	0.171	0.053
Personal Identity (Item 10: Hudson's PSSP)	0.186	0.217
Class III (low association expected)		
Age	−0.044	−0.077
Race	0.012	−0.018
Education	0.070	0.036
IQ (Full Scale)	−0.113	−0.107

sized to correlate highly with the Generalized Contentment Scale and the Index of Self-Esteem and were used as Class I values while the total PSSP scale score was used as a Class II (moderately correlating) value. In other words, a statement such as "I feel depressed" is expected to highly correlate with the Generalized Contentment Scale and Index of Self-Esteem while the PSSP's total score should only moderately associate with the GCS and ISE.

Findings. The guided self-rating method (described above) enabled 100% of the subjects (n = 75) to answer every item on each of the research scales. All of the instruments' internal reliability as tested by Cronbach's Alpha Coefficient is provided in Table 1. Three of the four self-rating instruments (GCS, ISE, and Rosenberg) and the two clinician observation scales (NSRS and PSAS) demonstrated moderately high stability. Only the Zung Depression Scale's reliability dropped to a low or questionable acceptability range. This was not altogether unexpected. Tanaka-Matsumi and Kameoka (1986) reported that when used with college students (n = 391) the Zung's alpha coefficient was only .81. Therefore, the .73 correlation found in this study may accurately reflect the instrument's internal consistency when used with extremely ill clients. Reliability based on a test-retest correlation for the Generalized Contentment Scale was .83 (p < .000) and .86 (p < .000) for the Index of Self-Esteem.

Concurrent instrument validity for the GCS was .88 and .91 for Hudson's ISE scale. A correlation matrix was used to measure the two Hudson scales' construct validity. Coefficients for the correlation by variable class are given in Table 2. A moderately high level of construct validity was found. As expected, the highest association occurred between the GCS and ISE themselves. A rather strong correlation, however, was also found among the Zung Depression Scale, GCS, and ISE. Only a moderate association occurred among the Rosenberg Self-Esteem Scale, GCS, and ISE. Furthermore, the Rosenberg unexpectedly associated slightly higher with the GCS than the ISE. The reverse had been anticipated. Perhaps more importantly and more concerning, the PSAS observer's depression rating (Table 2) had a rather low association with both the GCS and the ISE. The Hudson GCS indicated the clients had a much higher level of depressive symptoms than observed by the trained PSAS rater. Unfortunately, because one clinician performed the PSAS observations, an interrater reliability coefficient could not be calculated. As a result, it cannot be determined if the low correlation between the PSAS and GCS has any relevant clinical meaning. Nonetheless, this is an important question that must be addressed by future research. A valid instrument that definitively identifies depressive symptoms separately from negative symptoms in clients with schizophrenia is greatly needed.

Discussion. Poor concentration and similar negative symptoms make completing self-rating scales very difficult for severely mentally ill clients. Nonetheless, by using the clinician guided self-rating technique, individuals who had an extremely high level of psychotic and negative symptoms completed every item on each of the instruments. This was achieved largely because symptoms were differentially addressed, acknowledged, and accommodated for as the instruments were presented. As an example, time was always taken for labeling hallucinations, reassuring safety or confidentiality, and clarifying the instrument's purpose. Clients were also allowed to take short breaks and provide responses while pacing. The guided self-rating method places responsibility on the social worker for insuring a client's anxiety, frustration, or psychotic symptoms do not escalate unrecognized and undermine the assessment. That is, administering clinical scales to severely mentally ill clients requires one to identify and intervene with changing symptoms and attitudinal shifts before the measurement process is disrupted or invalidated.

Social workers may determine a client's need for momentarily delaying the self-rating exercise by observing minute changes in the individual's muscle tension; motor skills; eye movement; eye gaze and direction; sub-vocalization; speech pattern; attention and object of attention; cognitive processing speed and style; concentration; posture and body movement; or verbal tone and content. Many people with severe mental illness have random hallucinations throughout each day. The hallucinations may cause a person to stop attending to the assessment process and gaze to one side or another and focus on events occurring internally. At moments such as this the social worker may want to stop reading the scale item and softly acknowledge what is being clinically observed. This can be accomplished by simply asking the person, "Are you seeing or hearing something caused by your illness?" Obviously, this presumes the client is able and willing to acknowledge when hallucinations occur. After the client confirms the observation or offers an alternative perspective, the worker can provide supportive reassurance and ask the client to refocus on the assessment instrument. If the symptoms continue to escalate, the worker might suggest a short refreshment break or postpone the assessment.

The high level of reliability achieved by Hudson's GCS and ISE scales provides support for including the instruments when assessing clients with serious mental illness or evaluating treatment progress. Hudson reports alpha coefficients ranging from .89 to .96 for the GCS and between .91 and .95 for the ISE scale (Hudson, 1982; Abell, Jones, & Hudson, 1984). The SPMI population had reliability levels at or near the lower end of coefficients found by Hudson and associates for non-psychotic clients. Furthermore, time did not erode the reliability of the Hudson instruments studied with a test-retest model. After fourteen days the Generalized Contentment Scale and Index of Self-Esteem maintained a moderate level of internal consistency. An instrument with reliability of .80 or higher and psychometrically proven validity is generally considered acceptable for clinical assessments (Hudson, 1982).

The concurrent instrument validity findings indicate that the GCS, Zung Depression scale, and Hudson Index of Self-Esteem (ISE) measure similar responses (criterion). Likewise, the ISE and Rosenberg self-esteem items appear to identify highly-related perceptions. The pattern of intercorrelations between depression and self-esteem instruments strongly suggests that the scales, when used with this population, are measuring similar or identical factors. Therefore, the validity of the instruments for discretely measuring depression and self-esteem in clients with schizophrenia is not clear. The findings do, however, indicate that the scales are measuring responses that resemble depression and self-esteem factors in clients who have a psychosis. While this sounds like a play on words, it is psychometrically extremely important. The scales may indicate concurrent instrument validity because the criterion indicators are mislabeled. That is, when used with clients who have schizophrenia, the highly correlated responses may resemble, but in reality be accounting for, symptoms that have very little to do with depression and self-esteem. We must consider this as a possibility since in the past ten years neither the Zung nor Rosenberg has been validated with clients who have extremely severe schizophrenia symptoms.

Hudson (1984) found that the GCS and Zung had correlations ranging between .81 and .92. No known previous concurrent criterion validity coefficients for the ISE have been reported in the literature. To completely satisfy the question of concurrent instrument validity, the GCS and ISE need to be studied using the "known group" method. This is a method that requires expert clinicians to assign individuals with SPMI into high, medium, and low self-esteem or depression groups. Concurrent instrument validity is established if the GCS and ISE scale scores significantly differ among the groups and are directionally correct. In other words, knowing a client's score should increase the probability of predicting which symptom or diagnostic group (high, medium, or low) the individual was placed in by the expert judges.

Establishing construct validity for instruments measuring depression and self-esteem in clients with SPMI is complicated and difficult. Schizophrenia results from a damaged brain that creates positive and negative symptoms as well as incorrect perceptions of self and others (Taylor, 2003, 1987). Many individuals have schizophrenia and experience periods of depression. Correctly assessing whether both problems are concurrently present is difficult because negative symptoms "mock" depressive indicators. As a result, construct validity based on one relatively small homogeneous group must be viewed cautiously. Construct validity is indicated because Hudson's Generalized Contentment Scale and Index of Self-Esteem associate as predicted with variables ranked on a continuum. However, this should be considered a weak or heuristic finding until the results are replicated, and a concrete separation is made between negative symptoms and indicators that predict depression. The lack of association among IQ, education, GCS, or ISE supports current bio-psychosocial theories of schizophrenia, depression, and self-esteem. Furthermore, as expected, relatively high association levels were found among the GCS, ISE, Zung Depression scale, and Rosenberg Self-Esteem scores. Therefore, it would appear that all of these scales are measuring similar psychiatric problems.

One must wonder, however, if the high association between the GCS and ISE is because the two scales are measuring overlapping negative symptom constructs within the SPMI population. The unexpected small association among the Negative Symptoms Scale, GCS, and ISE may occur because the total scope of items within each scale is very different. Unlike the Negative Symptoms Scale, Hudson's depression and self-esteem instruments contain no items measuring a client's memory and concentration. Conversely, because of the close relationship between negative and depressive symptoms, the GCS and ISE may incorrectly weight scores for symptoms that are similar but nonetheless different from affective depression. Lower than predicted coefficients also occurred when PSAS observed depression and Hudson's PSSP self-rated self-esteem scores were correlated with the GCS and ISE. The PSAS scores may reflect the rater's: (a) need for additional training; (b) a bias toward rating depression and low self-esteem as negative symptoms; or (c) superior judgment of the clients' observable behaviors and symptoms. Additionally, it is also possible that the three instruments (PSAS, GCS, ISE) are measuring completely different theoretical constructs. These same psychometric concerns are equally true for the Psycho-Social Screening Package (PSSP) items.

Questions in the PSSP concerning self-esteem and depression are rather abstract. This forces a client to perform global information processing and develop a cognitive gestalt drawn from introspective perceptions. A high degree of frontal cortex brain functioning is required for performing this type of thinking (Torrey, 2001). An individual with schizophrenia most often has a damaged frontal cortex that processes cognitive cues more slowly and concretely than people with no history of psychosis (Taylor, 2003; Taylor, 1987; Torrey et al., 1994). Furthermore, self-esteem may be much more difficult to self-rate than depression. This would be particularly true if an individual had rapidly changing internal perceptions caused by anxiety. Additionally, people may have situational or social-contextual self-esteem rates that are influenced by ecological factors as well as a more constant internalized "trait" self-esteem level. These factors would make responding to a one dimensional self-esteem scale such as Hudson's ISE rather difficult for a client with schizophrenia.

LIMITATIONS

It is important to restate that this study consists of a non-randomized, small, homogeneous sample. Not only is generalization beyond the current population impossible but, in addition, reliability and validity of the scales with female and minority subjects who have SPMI were not adequately tested. Neurobiological illnesses also confound and cloud reliability and validity findings. As an example, a client may momentarily become fixated on a positive or negative perception that does not reflect good reality testing. Nonetheless, the perception may become part of the client's current belief system and structure the individual's responses to the scale items. Yet, in a short time period the cognitive perseveration or compulsion may disappear. How cognitive shifts impact self-rating scales can only be understood when the research design includes multiple systematic measurements over an extended time period. This study consists of only two measurement points fourteen days apart. Furthermore, a scale's reliability and validity can only be established when agreement is found among numerous replicated studies.

The guided self-rating system created for helping SPMI clients focus and complete the rating scales also presents a psychometric problem. The researcher made every effort not to prompt and bias the client's responses. A system was put in place to insure that the researcher did not review clinical notes, previous psychological testing, or attend treatment oriented meetings to discuss the client's psychiatric status before the self-rating scales were administered. Nevertheless, until reliability and validity are shown to remain stable across multiple trained clinicians (using the guided self-rating method), researcher bias must be considered.

CONCLUSION

This study demonstrates that when a guided self-rating method is employed, severely mentally ill clients can reliably complete clinical assessment instruments. Therefore, short psychometrically valid scales may provide an economical and meaningful tool for case managers to monitor their clients' symptoms, medication responses, and psychosocial functioning. Hudson's General Contentment and Index of Self-Esteem scales reflected almost the same level of reliability reported for non-psychotic clients. Additionally, the General Contentment Scale had more reliability when used with clients who have extremely severe symptoms than the more traditional Zung Depression Scale. Furthermore, within the limitations of this study, it was found that the Hudson instruments might have a modest level of concurrent criterion and construct validity. However, validity was established strictly from a heuristic research perspective and does not provide support for clinical interpretations of scale scores. All of the study's findings must be seen as preliminary and greatly in need of replication before social workers can interpret the clinical scores with confidence.

The results of this study are encouraging considering the participants were extremely ill and continuously disrupted by positive and negative symptoms. Individuals with more controlled or mild symptoms may not require the guided self-rating method for completing the scales. Unfortunately, measuring how differing levels of illness severity affect the instruments' psychometric qualities was beyond this study's scope. Currently, social workers are cautiously encouraged to use the GCS and ISE scales for evaluating symptom intensity, treatment or program effectiveness, and client perceptual changes. The reliability of these scales with extremely ill clients may allow clinicians to identify symptom shifts even though the exact underlying construct being measured remains uncertain. Until further research is conducted, the instruments are not seen as helpful nor are they recommended for initial assessments with individuals who have serious mental illness. The scores, when collaborated with other independent assessment methods, can help guide treatment recommendations. In addition, the Hudson GCS and ISE can be used to establish reliable baselines for tracking possible affective symptoms and help signal to clinicians when emergency treatment planning is needed to deal with unexpectedly escalating symptoms placing a client at risk for suicide.

REFERENCES

Abell, N., Jones, B.L., & Hudson, W.W. (1984). Revalidation of the index of self-esteem. *Social Work Research and Abstracts, 20*, 11-16.

Bigelow, L., & Berthot, B.D. (1989). The psychiatric symptom assessment scale (PSAS). *Psychopharmacology Bulletin, 25*,168-179.

Black, D.W., & Andreasen, N.C. (1999). Schizophrenia, and schizophreniform disorder, and delusional (paranoid) disorders. In Robert E. Hales, Stuart C. Yudofsky, & John A. Talbott (Eds.), *Textbook of Psychiatry, 3rd Ed*. Washington, DC: American Psychiatric Press, pp. 425-478.

Grebb, J.A., Shelton, R.C., Taylor, E.H., & Bigelow, L.B. (1986). A negative, double-blind, placebo-controlled, clinical trial of Verapamil in chronic schizophrenia. *Biological Psychiatry, 21*, 691-694.

Hale, D., & Hale, R.E. (1995). *Caring for the Mind: The Comprehensive Guide to Mental Health*. New York: Bantam Books.

Hudson, W.W. (1982). *The Clinical Measurement Package: A Field Manual*. Homewood, IL: The Dorsey Press.

Jaeger, A.C., Kirch, D.G., & Wyatt, R.J. (1986). Negative symptom rating scale. *Psychiatry Research, 19*, 171-173.

Nicole, L., & Shriqui, C.L. (1995). Gender differences in schizophrenia. In Christian L. Shriqui & Henry A. Nasrallah (Eds.), *Contemporary Issues in the Treatment of Schizophrenia*. Washington, DC: American Psychiatric Press, pp. 225-243.

Nunnally, J.C., & Bernstein, I.H. (1994). *Psychometric Theory, third edition*. New York: McGraw-Hill.

Overall, J.E., & Gorham, D.R. (1962). The brief psychiatric rating scale. *Psychological Reports, 10*, 799-812.

Rosenberg, M. (1965). *Society and the Adolescent Self-Image*. Princeton: Princeton University Press.

Tanaka-Matsumi, J., & Kameoka, V.A. (1986). Reliabilities and concurrent validities of popular self-report measures of depression, anxiety, and social desirability. *Journal of Consulting & Clinical Psychology, 54*, 328-333.

Taylor, E.H. (2003). Practice methods for working with children who have biologically based disorders: A bioecological model. *Families and Society.*

Taylor, E.H. (2002). Manic depression. In V.S. Ramachandran (Ed.), *Encyclopedia of the Human Brain, Vol. 2.* San Diego: Academic Press, 745-757.

Taylor, E.H. (1987). The biological basis of schizophrenia. *Social Work, 32,* 115-121.

Torrey, E.F. (2001). *Surviving Schizophrenia.* New York: Quill.

Torrey, E.F., Bowler, A.E., Taylor, E.H., & Gottesman, I.I. (1994). *Schizophrenia and Manic Depressive Disorder: The Biological Roots of Mental Illness as Revealed by the Landmark Study of Identical Twins.* New York: Basic Books.

Zung, W.K. (1965). A self-rating depression scale. *Archives of General Psychiatry, 12,* 63-70.

APPENDIX

Clinical Administration of the Guided Self-Rating Method

The guided self-rating method requires the clinician to read each question aloud and record the client's verbal response. The following protocol was followed for all subjects:

- participant was assured that no reading is required;
- a single rating scale was shown and fully explained;
- the scale was placed on a table in front of the participant, and all scale items were covered with a blank sheet of paper;
- the scale responses (i.e., responses for Hudson scales = (1) Rarely or none of the time; (2) A little of the time; (3) Some of the time, etc.) were pointed out and read one by one exactly as they appear on the scale;
- each scale item was individually uncovered (all other items remained covered by blank sheet of paper) and read to the participant;
- the researcher then asked, "Which of these (pointing to the scale responses) best answers this item for you? Let's review the choices again. Is this true: rarely or none of the time; a little of the time; some of the time; a good part of the time; or most or all of the time?";
- the participant's selected response was recorded in the provided space by the researcher;
- the forced-choice responses were reread after each item until the participant indicated it was not required and independently selected one of the forced choice responses.

When a participant's concentration was broken by hallucinations or other symptoms, the researcher acknowledged the difficulty, allowed a short break (1-5 minutes without leaving the table), and then repeated the uncompleted scale item. Upon finishing a scale the client and researcher would take a short walk and engage in friendly non-clinical conversation.

Assessing Tradition in Chinese Elders Living in a Changing Social Environment: Implications for Social Work Practice

Lee Ann Mjelde-Mossey
Iris Chi
Vivian W. Q. Lou

SUMMARY. Social workers are increasingly challenged to provide culturally sensitive services to older immigrants from diverse backgrounds. Assessment tools developed in the elder's own cultural context can maximize appropriate assessment and planning. This article describes the development of a tool for measuring adherence to tradition in Chinese elders. In Chinese tradition, an elder's purpose, meaning, and self-worth are derived, in large part, from their contribution to family,

Lee Ann Mjelde-Mossey, PhD, MSW, is Assistant Professor, College of Social Work, the Ohio State University, Columbus, OH and Research Fellow, Sau Po Centre on Aging, The University of Hong Kong.

Iris Chi, DSW, is Professor, Department of Social Work and Social Administration and Director, Sau Po Centre on Aging, University of Hong Kong, Pokfulam Road, Hong Kong (E-mail: irischi@hku.hk). Vivian W. Q. Lou, PhD, is Research Associate, Sau Po Centre on Aging, University of Hong Kong (E-mail: wlou@hkucc.hku.hk).

Address correspondence to: Lee Ann Mjelde-Mossey, PhD, MSW, Assistant Professor, College of Social Work, the Ohio State University, 1947 College Road, Columbus, OH 43210-1162 (E-mail: mjelde-mossey.1@osu.edu).

[Haworth co-indexing entry note]: "Assessing Tradition in Chinese Elders Living in a Changing Social Environment: Implications for Social Work Practice." Mjelde-Mossey, Lee Ann, Iris Chi, and Vivian W. Q. Lou. Co-published simultaneously in *Journal of Human Behavior in the Social Environment* (The Haworth Social Work Practice Press, an imprint of The Haworth Press, Inc.) Vol. 11, No. 3/4, 2005, pp. 41-57; and: *Approaches to Measuring Human Behavior in the Social Environment* (ed: William R. Nugent) The Haworth Social Work Practice Press, an imprint of The Haworth Press, Inc., 2005, pp. 41-57. Single or multiple copies of this article are available for a fee from The Haworth Document Delivery Service [1-800-HAWORTH, 9:00 a.m. - 5:00 p.m. (EST). E-mail address: docdelivery@haworthpress.com].

Available online at http://www.haworthpress.com/web/JHBSE
doi:10.1300/J137v11n03_03

relatives, and the community. Existing measures of filial piety and acculturation do not capture this dimension. Filial piety involves being on the receiving end of care, honor, and obedience from younger generations. Acculturation is the opposite of adherence to tradition. One thousand five-hundred and two Chinese elders in China were asked questions on mutual aid and intergenerational exchange. Factor analysis extracted nine items loading into two factors reflective of traditional exchange. This measure could prove useful in understanding the effect of traditional beliefs upon various psychosocial outcomes. *[Article copies available for a fee from The Haworth Document Delivery Service: 1-800-HAWORTH. E-mail address: <docdelivery@haworthpress.com> Website: <http://www.HaworthPress.com> © 2005 by The Haworth Press, Inc. All rights reserved.]*

KEYWORDS. Tradition, culture, assessment, Chinese, aged

The majority of older Chinese in the United States are immigrants. According to the 2000 U.S. Census, 60.6% of Asian-Americans of all ages, and 71.0% of Asian- and Pacific Islander-Americans over age 65, are foreign-born (He, 2002). These demographics make it imperative for helping professionals to be sensitive to traditions that guide norms, values, expectations, attitudes, and behaviors in those who lived most of their life in another culture. This article looks specifically at Chinese traditional culture and older adults and seeks to describe how adherence to tradition in that age group might be measured. Existing measures of filial piety and acculturation do not tap into this dimension, most likely because of a limited Western understanding of Chinese culture. While both filial piety and acculturation provide very useful information, neither reflects the worldview of an elder who spent the majority of his or her life immersed in, and adhering to, an ancient culture. Measuring acculturation in particular reflects a Western bias because higher levels of change from indigenous to Western culture are usually considered positive. This article suggests that, when evaluating a Chinese elder, cultural sensitivity must include an understanding of the elder's worldview and how it might exacerbate a problem or, hopefully, contribute to a solution. Green (1998) describes cultural sensitivity in a multi-ethnic society as being open, alert, accepting, and flexible in relations with clients from diverse backgrounds. Other helping professionals go so far as to say that it is not possible to understand another person without clearly understanding his/her traditional base (Ivey, Ivey, and Simek-Morgan, 1997; Sue, Ivey, and Pedersen, 1996). More specifically, Duan and Wang (2000) proposed that, by not considering cultural demands, any lasting and effective change for Chinese clients could be precluded. It follows, then, that helping professionals can benefit from accepting the notion of individual worldviews. A worldview can be described as the ways that a person perceives his/her self in relation to the world and how those perceptions affect thoughts, decisions, behavior, and interpretation of events (Sue, 1981). Thus, developing a measure of tradition, from the perspective of the older person, could prove useful to understanding the relationship between adherence to tradition and various psychosocial outcomes.

CHINESE TRADITION AND AGING

Chinese culture has been described as a high-context culture. An individual in this culture is part of an extended network of family and kin relationships. In addition, traditionally, the family and kin usually live in close proximity to each other. Thus, the individual's self and self-worth is connected to others through well-established and well-understood commitments, loyalties, rights, and responsibilities (Hall, 1983). Within this context, the centrality of family for Chinese elders cannot be overstated. Elders depend upon younger generations for both emotional and instrumental support. Because of this dependence, the concept of filial piety is often understood in Western cultures to be primarily the obligation of the young to provide for their parents. There is more to filial piety and, based in Confucianism, it also includes honoring and obeying elders. In this way one honors one's ancestors and brings honor to the greater community as well (Ho, 1996). Although filial piety is the building block of family relations, Chinese elders are expected to be contributors to the well-being of the family and community. Giving advice, comforting, teaching, and helping others in need are vital to proper behavior for Chinese elders. For a Chinese elder, caring for grandchildren is not an act of "babysitting"; it is a cultural imperative. In the pure Chinese tradition of *xiao*, or filial piety, elders are expected to play a meaningful role in both family and society and thus ensure harmony with nature, others, and even themselves (Chow, 1999). The guiding principle for these social behaviors for maintaining harmony is known as *Renqing* or social exchanges based upon giving rather than receiving (Cheung et al., 1996). These networks of exchanges and the positive meaning attached to giving were essential to basic survival in the past. In times when the nuclear family could not help, it was expected that those who were able would provide assistance to those in need (Xiangqun, 1999). So, while Westerners attempt to understand Chinese elders based upon how much help their children give them, or how much of their culture they have shed, the very essence of what underpins quality of life and self-worth for Chinese elders is missed, that of being a contributing member of the social group. Traditional Chinese elders are defined by the collective and their purpose, meaning, and self-worth are derived from how positively they affect the group and by their contribution to the collective. Thus, their contribution helps to maintain harmony in the family which, in turn, contributes to harmony in the community and, ultimately, to an orderly universe (Chow, 1996).

Western Theories of Social Exchange

In the Western literature, the two dominant theoretical perspectives on intergenerational exchange and family relationships are social exchange theory and equity theory. It is quite likely that a Chinese elder could be misunderstood if these theoretical frameworks were applied. In fact, these theories of social exchange and their relationship to well-being may highlight differences between aging in Western and Chinese cultures. Social exchange theory is based upon the idea that social exchange and interaction will continue only as long as benefits are seen to outweigh the costs (Cook, 1987; Thibaut and Kelley, 1959). In social exchange theory, the purpose of social relationships is self-serving and will be maintained for as long as one is getting more than they give. Social exchanges are based upon rational choice and behavior is not influenced by cultural and social environments (Homans, 1958). Equity theory proposes that relationships are most satisfactory when giving and getting are perceived as being about equal. This balance of giving and receiving means that a person would be dissatisfied with relationships in which they give more than they receive (Walster, Walster, and Berscheid, 1978; Feeney, Peterson, and Noller, 1994). Neither of these theories captures the meaning of social exchanges for traditional Chinese elders.

There is a theory of human behavior that could be applied to this study. Based upon symbolic interaction, the social constructionist perspective posits that people learn to understand the world, and their place in it, through their interactions with others (Stryker, 1980). An individual will form beliefs about their worth from social interactions and these beliefs will shape their subsequent social interactions. In this perspective, people are seen as social beings who interact with each other based upon shared meanings and understanding of the world. However, while the social constructionist perspective may closely describe how behaviors are learned, it does not give weight or value to those behaviors.

METHOD

Participants and Sampling

Participants were recruited from randomly selected counties within three randomly selected newly-developed towns near Beijing, Guangzhou, and Shanghai. Newly-developed towns are geographic areas contiguous to large urban cities and have transitioned from rural farms and villages to urban environments during the last decade. Thus, a newly developed town is one that was defined as a suburb area (village) before 1992 but became urbanized after 1994. New towns are also characterized by replacement of the traditional village with high-rise apartments. In this situation, families that lived in villages or farms for generations lost their lifestyle, community networks, and utilization of the land when they officially re-registered their residence from rural to urban (Pu, Chen, and Zhou, 1995). This changing social environment may parallel the experience of immigrating to a Western culture.

The elders recruited for this study were selected from a list of residents provided by the local statistics bureau in the three new towns. Those who met the criteria of being age 60 or over and had transitioned from rural to urban qualified for the study. About 500 participants were randomly selected from each new town. Random replacement was made for those in the original cohort who could not participate due to language, travel, elected not to, or did not fully complete the questionnaire. The age range of the sample was 60 to 94 years with a mean of 69.7 and standard deviation of 6.8. Of the 1,502 participants, 61.2% were female and 38.8% were male; 59.5% were married; 31.9% had formal education; 88.9% lived with others; 45.3% rated their health from "good" to "excellent"; and 80.7% rated their financial adequacy from "just enough" to "more than adequate." See Table 1 for more detail on characteristics of the sample.

Data Collection

After the selection process was completed, county representatives contacted the elders and introduced the purpose of the study. Prospective participants were asked if they would agree to be interviewed. If the response was affirmative, the county representative and the elder set a date and time when the interview would take place. The interviews were conducted by college students who were given intensive training and close supervision. Each interview took an average of 60 minutes to complete. The questionnaire included items on demographic characteristics, health and functioning, finances, social networks, service utilization, service needs, mood, and life satisfaction. Each of the completed questionnaires was reviewed by a project supervisor. If a questionnaire had more than 20% missing data it was excluded from the analysis and random replacement was made for more interviews. As a result, 1,502 elders were successfully interviewed within a three-month period. The final data set included 500 each from the new towns in Guangzhou and Shanghai and 502 from Beijing.

Questions on Tradition

The questionnaire included items on family relations, intergenerational exchange and social networks. Nine items reflective of tradi-

TABLE 1. Sample Characteristics

	Frequency (%)			
n	Shanghai (500)	Beijing (502)	Guangzhou (500)	Total (1,502)
Sex				
Male	154 (30.8)	211 (42.0)	218 (43.6)	583 (38.8)
Female	346 (69.2)	291 (58.0)	282 (56.4)	919 (61.2)
Age				
60-64	134 (26.8)	153 (30.5)	117 (23.4)	404 (26.9)
65-69	119 (23.8)	137 (27.3)	128 (25.6)	384 (25.6)
70-74	110 (22.0)	113 (22.5)	132 (26.4)	355 (23.6)
75 or above	137 (27.4)	99 (19.7)	123 (24.6)	359 (23.9)
Formal education				
Yes	185 (37.0)	129 (25.7)	65 (33.0)	479 (31.9)
No	315 (63.0)	373 (74.3)	335 (67.0)	1,023 (68.1)
Marital status				
Currently married	318 (63.6)	308 (61.4)	267 (53.4)	893 (59.5)
Currently not married	182 (36.4)	194 (38.6)	233 (46.6)	609 (40.5)

tional relationships, beliefs, values, or behaviors were selected for factor analysis. All nine of the questions were answered either "agree" or "disagree."

Four of the items related to an elder's income and financial aid. One question, "children should take responsibility for the financial need of the elderly" is a clear statement of filial piety. Two of the questions, "receive financial assistance from children when in need" and "seek help from children on financial difficulties" indicate that children either provide financial aid or the elder would turn to children in times of financial need. The last question, "source of income from children" is indicative of actual income support from children. Questions about income and financial aid are considered highly representative of Chinese tradition. Of the three cornerstones of filial piety, i.e., honor, obey, and care for, the most dominant remnant of that tradition is financial support of parents. Even if younger generations no longer ask for permission or blindly accept an elder's advice, they do generally continue to provide income support. This is particularly true for contemporary elders whose children may no longer live in close proximity to them (Chan and Leong, 1994).

Two other questions touched upon the honor and care aspects of filial piety. "Other people talk to you for important decisions" is highly reflective of honoring the wisdom of elders and reflects the importance of age and experience in offering guidance to others. Lastly, a question asked if children could be counted on to provide care when the elder was ill.

Three items on giving social and instrumental support to others captured this very important and lesser known aspect of Chinese tradition. It is by giving to others that elders help to ensure balance and harmony in the family, community, and universe (Chow, 1999). Two questions asked about giving "comfort" to immediate family or extended relatives "when they feel down." Giving comfort is, qualitatively, very different from giving advice. Comforting others does not imply drawing upon an elder's wisdom, rather, it is a form of affective giving that is altruistic and non-obligatory. It is also important to note that comfort is given outside of the immediate family circle. Ho (1986) mentioned the importance of elders giving affective support in the traditional Chinese community. The third question asked the elder if he/she "helps people around with household tasks." This question also reflects the elder's contribution to the family and the community. In the Western concept of Chinese elders, there is a tendency to conceptualize Chinese elders as being passive recipients of instrumental aid, when, in reality, elders derive much of their self-worth from being contributing members of the family and community (Yang, 1995).

Data Analysis

All the statistical analysis was performed using SPSS (SPSS, Inc., 1999). Scale reliability and factor analysis for the tradition measure were conducted first. Answers to the nine factored items were dummy coded as agree = 1 and disagree = 0. Varimax rotation and the principle component method were used to extract items that loaded into factors. Varimax was chosen because it is thought to be the conservative approach in the formulation of a new measure. Internal consistency of the entire scale and subscales was computed as indicated by Cronbach's alpha. For the final measure of tradition, each of the nine items was given equal weight. The higher an individual scored, the higher his/her level of tradition. In this sample, the range of scores was from 0 to 9 with a mean of 5.15 and standard deviation of 2.20. The responses ranged from 22.2% (n = 333) for "comfort extended relatives when they feel down" to 79.4% (n = 1,193) for "count on children when you are ill." The frequency distribution of the nine items is presented in Table 2.

An ANOVA method was used to assess for differences in socio-demographic variables and associated levels of tradition. Tukey HSD was used to test Post Hoc differences in variables with more than two values. Age was divided into four categories (60-64 = 1, 65-69 = 2, 70-74 = 3, 75 and above = 4). Married, formal education, living alone, and living with children were coded yes = 1 and no = 0. Kruskal-Wallis and

TABLE 2. Frequency Distribution of the Items

	Agree (%) (N = 1,502)
Count on children when you are ill	1,193 (79.4)
Seek help from children on financial difficulties	1,125 (74.9)
Children should take responsibility for financial needs of elderly	1,075 (71.6)
Source of income from children	945 (62.9)
Help people around with household tasks	847 (56.4)
Receive financial assistance from children when in need	774 (51.5)
Comfort immediate family members when they feel down	752 (50.1)
Other people talk to you for important decision	690 (41.9)
Comfort extended relatives when they feel down	333 (22.2)

Spearman r were also used to test for relationships in the ordinal variables of self-rated health, self-rated financial adequacy, and working status due to concerns about normality assumptions when ANOVA is used with ordinal data. Working status was entered as four categories of currently employed, currently non-employed, retired, and homemaker/never-employed. Self-rated health was assessed by a single item question, "how would you rate your overall health at this time?" on a five-point scale (1 = poor, 2 = fair, 3 = good, 4 = very good, 5 = excellent). Self-rated health is a valid and reliable measure of health status (Ferraro and Kelley-Moore, 2001; Pijls, Feskens, and Kromhout, 1993). Financial adequacy was also measured by a single item question, "do you think that you have enough money to cover your daily expenses?" on a three-point scale (1 = less than adequate, 2 = just enough, 3 = more than adequate).

Tradition scores for each of the new towns were also compared in the ANOVA as an anchor for the other variables. This is one of the benefits of having data from three separate new towns that are known to have regional differences in tradition (Deng, 2000; Wu, 2002; Xie et al., 1997; Zhao et al., 1998). The three regional areas known as Hua Bei (North), Hua Dong (East), and Hua Nan (South) are where Beijing, Shanghai, and Guangzhou are located respectively. Of the three locations, Beijing is considered to be the most traditional. Beijing is land-bound as well as the capital of China and, therefore, very closely connected to tradition and comparatively slow to change. Shanghai is a major seaport, with interests in international trade and finance, and considered to be the least traditional. In fact, Shanghai is considered to be the most Westernized city in China with a reputation for openness and tolerance of cultural diversity (Li, 2002; Zhang, 2002).

RESULTS

Tradition Scale Development

Varimax rotation and principle component method extracted nine items that loaded into two factors. Internal consistency was satisfactory with a Cronbach's alpha for the total scale of .67. The Cronbach's alpha for factor one was .69 and .61 for factor two. An eigenvalue larger than one was the criterion for retaining a factor. The total scale explained 45.8% of the variance. Factor one, which included four items on receiving financial assistance from children, explained 23.9% of the variance.

Factor two, which included five items on giving or receiving instrumental and social support (mutual aid), explained 21.9% of the variance. Table 3 gives more detail on the rotated factor loadings.

Group Differences on Tradition

Results of the ANOVA testing for significant differences in tradition scores within the socio-demographic variables and new towns of residence are presented in Table 4. Those living in Beijing scored highest on mean scores on tradition (5.97), Guangzhou was next (5.54), and Shanghai had the lowest mean scores (3.94) which proved to be significantly different (F = 140.07, p < .001). Of the remaining nine variables, all but gender were found to have significantly different mean scores. Even though females were found to have higher scores on tradition, the difference was not statistically significant (F = 2.09, p > .05). Mean scores by age category were significantly different, particularly between those who were 75 and older and those younger (F = 14.96, p < .001). Those who were age 75 and older scored lowest on tradition. Regarding working status, those who were homemaker/never employed

TABLE 3. Rotated Factor Loadings

	Factor 1	Factor 2
Receive financial assistance from children when in need	**.75**	.11
Source of income from children	**.73**	.01
Children should take responsibility for financial needs of elderly	**.69**	.01
Seek help from children on financial difficulties	**.68**	.01
Comfort immediate family members when they feel down	.14	**.78**
Comfort extended relatives when they feel down	.01	**.69**
Other people talk to you for important decision	.01	**.67**
Help people around with household tasks	.01	**.53**
Count on children when you are ill	.30	**.36**
Cronbach's alpha	.69	.61
Initial Eigenvalues	2.52	1.60
Variance Explained (%)	23.9	21.9
Cumulative %	45.8	
Total Cronbach's alpha	.67	

TABLE 4. Characteristics and Group Differences on Tradition

	Tradition Mean (SD)	F (df)	Post-Hoc Tukey	KW χ^2 (df)	Spearman r
Sex					
Male	5.05 (2.17)	2.09	NIL		
Female	5.21 (2.22)	(1,1500)			
Age					
60-64 (1)[a]	5.39 (2.20)	14.96***	1/4[b]		
65-69 (2)	5.39 (2.14)	(3,1498)	2/4		
70-74 (3)	5.29 (2.08)		3/4		
75 or above (4)	4.48 (2.24)				
Working status				18.1	.05*
Currently employed (1)	5.31 (2.34)	5.60***	3/4	(3)	
Currently non-employed (2)	5.64 (2.41)	(3,1498)			
Retired (3)	5.04 (2.20)				
Homemaker/ never employed (4)	5.73 (2.01)				
Formal education					
Yes	4.95 (2.20)	5.56*	NIL		
No	5.24 (2.19)	(1,1500)			
Marital status					
Currently married	5.32 (2.12)	13.46***	NIL		
Currently not married	4.90 (2.29)	(1,1500)			
Living alone					
Yes	3.73 (2.35)	82.53***	NIL		
No	5.33 (2.11)	(1,1500)			
Living with children					
Yes	5.63 (1.99)	103.64***	NIL		
No	4.51 (2.29)	(1,1500)			
City					
Beijing (1)	5.97 (1.90)	140.07***	1/2,3		
Guangzhou (2)	5.54 (2.22)	(2,1499)	2/1,3		
Shanghai (3)	3.94 (1.92)				
Self-rated health				36	.15**
Poor (1)	4.62 (2.15)	8.91**	1/2,3,4,5	(4)	
Fair (2)	5.06 (2.20)	(4,1494)	2/1,5		
Good (3)	5.32 (2.09)		3/1		
Very good (4)	5.43 (2.18)		4/1		
Excellent (5)	5.65 (2.24)		5/1,2		
Self-rated financial adequacy				69.9	.22**
Less than adequate (1)	4.41 (2.12)	35.71***	1/2,3	(2)	
Just enough (2)	5.07 (2.18)	(2,1497)	2/1,3		
More than adequate (3)	5.75 (2.11)				

Notes: [a](1) (2) (3) (4) indicated group number as shown in the column under "Post-Hoc Tukey"
[b]significant difference was found between group 1 and 4, similar interpretation for other presentations in this column.
NIL = not applicable for Post-Hoc Tukey test
*p < .05, **p < .01, ***p < .001

scored higher on tradition compared to those having employment experiences but the difference was statistically significant for retired only ($F = 5.60$, $p < .01$). Those with no formal education scored significantly higher on tradition than those with formal education ($F = 5.56$, $p < .01$). Currently married elders had significantly higher tradition scores than those who were not currently married (including widowed, divorced, or separated) ($F = 13.46$, $p < .001$). Both of the living arrangement variables had significantly different scores, with those living with others ($F = 82.53$, $p < .001$) and those living with children ($F = 103.64$, $p < .001$) scoring higher on tradition. Elders who rated themselves in poor health had the lowest mean tradition scores. Categories of self-rated health were significantly different, with those who perceived themselves as healthier also scoring higher on tradition ($F = 8.91$, $p < .01$). There were significant differences in the mean tradition scores and self-ratings of financial adequacy, with those with higher finance ratings having higher tradition scores ($F = 35.71$, $p < .001$).

The nonparametric tests on the ordinal variables verified the ANOVA results. Kruskal-Wallis tests supported group differences in the ordinal variables of self-rated health ($\chi^2 = 36.0$, $df = 4$); self-rated financial adequacy ($\chi^2 = 69.9$, $df = 2$); and working status ($\chi^2 = 18.1$, $df = 3$). All three were significant at a better than $p < .005$, which supports that the groups were not the same. The Spearman rho was not very strong for any variable, but all were significant. Self-rated financial adequacy was the strongest with $r = .22$, self-rated health was weaker with $r = .15$, while working status was very weak with $r = .05$. See Table 4.

In summary, elders who scored significantly higher on tradition shared some characteristics. The more traditional elders were more likely to be younger, married, living with others or their children, have no formal education, be a never-employed homemaker, have better self-rated health and financial adequacy, and live in Beijing.

DISCUSSION

The significant differences in the mean scores of tradition in the new town variable bore out the regional differences between the new towns. This provides credence as well as insight into the measure and helps support the need for further exploration of a tradition construct. The idea of measuring Chinese tradition has other proponents who suggest that there is a dimension of personality variation called the "Chinese Tradition" (Bond, 2000; Zhang and Bond, 1998). For now, it is important to examine the two factors resulting from the factor analysis and discuss whether or not they are consistent with Chinese tradition.

Factor one is a clear statement of the tradition of filial piety in the form of children providing financial support to parents. Three of the items indicate that children provide financial aid in times of need or difficulties and children are a source of income for the elders. The fourth item indicates that elders retain the traditional expectation that children are responsible for the financial support of their parents. This expectation is as old as the saying of Confucius that "the fundamental principle was filial piety and the practice of support of parents" (Gernet, 1982, p. 159). The mean tradition scores reported in Table 4 lend conceptual support to this factor. Those scoring higher on tradition also reported they were currently not employed, had no formal education, and were homemaker/never employed, and presumably more likely to have financial need.

Factor two provides an interesting mix of filial piety and the other aspect of traditional old age: that of giving to others. Although the items may not seem to relate to each other, they really do describe traditional mutual aid between the elder, their family and the community. It is this interplay that can be overlooked or misunderstood when assessing a Chinese elder. Giving of themselves through helping others with social and instrumental support is a highly important part of a Chinese elder's role and image. The factor is also reflective of *Renqing* which is the underpinning principle for maintaining harmony in social relationships (Cheung et al., 1996). In addition, there is emerging evidence that giving social support has protective health benefits for the giver (Liang, Krause, and Bennet, 2001). Chinese elders may also empower themselves and develop a sense of inner strength through connection with others (Mok, 2001). The mean tradition scores reported in Table 4 lend conceptual support to this factor. Those scoring higher on tradition reported involvement with others in their social environment. Elders who lived with children, lived with others, or were currently married had higher tradition scores.

Looking at the significant differences in the mean tradition scores, the more traditional elders were more likely to be younger. This was an unexpected result but, upon closer examination, this cohort effect does connect to Chinese history. After the emergence of Sun Yat Sen and his alliance with Communist doctrines during the 1920s, the 1930s were a time when China's citizens were encouraged to focus on the future and discard the traditions of the past. This shift away from tradition culminated in the Cultural Revolution of the 1960s. The oldest participants in our study were heavily influenced by these events and known to be more liberal than younger cohorts of Chinese who became disenchanted with modernism and reverted to tradition (Hon, 1996).

The finding that genders did not have significantly different scores on tradition was also unexpected. Traditionally, women are responsible for teaching younger generations as well as passing on and maintaining social rituals and social networks (Xiangqun, 1999). Women did score higher, it just was not significant. Never employed homemakers and those with no formal education had significantly higher scores on tradition which seems consistent with persons who have less exposure to other cultures or ways of living. Elders who were presently married and living with others or their children, had significantly higher scores and this would emphasize the collective nature of Chinese tradition. Higher scores on tradition for those with self-rated financial adequacy could reflect the traditional practice of receiving financial aid and income from children. The result that those with higher scores on tradition have better self-rated health does not seem to relate to tradition in one way or the other. This finding would bear closer examination in a subsequent study.

Strengths and Limitations of the Study

While the limitations of this study are apparent, there are also considerable strengths. The main strength is that the results give direction to the next step of research designed specifically to refine and test a measure of tradition for older Chinese. This step should also include cross-national comparisons with immigrants living in other countries. Another strength is that it contributes to the cultural sensitivity of helping professionals in an area that is not well-known to Western practitioners. The main limitation of this study is that the questions used in the analysis were culled from a large study that was not focused on tradition. This limited our ability to factor a wider number of items.

Implications for Practice

The insights provided by this study of Chinese elders living in a changing social environment could parallel the experience of Chinese elders who have emigrated to a new society. Older Chinese immigrants to the United States tend to relocate to urban environments characterized by ethnic restaurants, shops, and activities that are within walking distances and where Chinese is the spoken language. In these urban enclaves, traditional beliefs and behaviors tend to be maintained and exert influence upon adaptation to a new culture. To add to that, older immigrants come with longer exposure to tradition which means that traditional beliefs, values and practices are more ingrained. It is important to consider these converging influences when trying to understand a Chinese elder. Gauging a Chinese elder's level of acculturation, or adaptation, to Western culture often presumes that higher levels of acculturation are more positive. Yet, in practice with a Chinese elder who is experiencing problems, any effort to Westernize their behavior, beliefs, or values may be the most counter-productive approach. For a traditional Chinese, behaving as one "should" contributes to harmony, honors ancestors, and brings good fortune. Attempts to override this belief system will probably not be successful. Instead, reframing traditional expectations in the context of the elder's current lifestyle could prove effective. For example, an elder may have problems with more acculturated adult children who perceive the elder's advice-giving as meddling or controlling. Family members can be empowered to draw upon personal strengths in which multiple worldviews and values of individual members are recognized, incorporated, and negotiated (Lee and Mjelde-Mossey, in press). It is hoped that the study reported here will give clearer understanding and direction to social work practice with Chinese elders.

REFERENCES

Bond, M.H. (2000). Localizing the imperial outreach: The Big Five and more in Chinese culture. *The American Behavioral Scientist*, 44, 63-72.

Chan, S., & Leong, C.W. (1994). Chinese families in transition: Cultural conflicts and adjustment problems. *Journal of Social Distress & the Homeless*, 3, 363-381.

Cheung, F.M.C., Leung, K., Fan, R., Song, W.Z., Zhang, J.X., & Zhang, J.P. (1996). Development of the Chinese personality assessment inventory. *Journal of Cross-Cultural Psychology*, 27, 181-199.

Chow, N.W.S. (1996). Filial piety in Asian Chinese communities. *Hong Kong Journal of Gerotonlogy*, 10 (Supplement), 115-117.

Chow, N.W.S. (1999). Diminishing filial piety and the changing role and status of the elders in Hong Kong. *Hallym International Journal of Aging*, 1, 67-77.

Cook, K. (1987). *Social exchange theory*. Newbury Park, CA: Sage Publications.

Deng, W. (2000). Contrastive analysis of death standards in Guangzhou, Beijing, and Shanghai. *South China Population*, 15, 19-24.

Duan, C., & Wang, L. (2000). Counseling in the Chinese cultural context: Accommodating both individualistic and collectivistic values. *Asian Journal of Counseling*, 7, 1-22.

Feeney, J., Peterson, C., & Noller, P. (1994). Equity and marital satisfaction over the family life cycle. *Personal Relationships*, 1, 83-99.

Ferraro, K.F., & Kelley-Moore, J.A. (2001). Self-rated health and mortality among black and white adults: Examining the dynamic evaluation thesis. *Journal of Gerontology: Social Sciences*, 56B, S195-S205.

Gernet, J. (1982). *A History of Chinese civilization* (2nd ed.). Cambridge, UK: Cambridge University Press.

Green, J.W. (1998). *Cultural awareness in the human services: A multi-ethnic approach* (3rd ed.). Needham Heights, MA: Allyn & Bacon.

Hall, E.T. (1983). *The Dance of Life*. Garden City, NY: Doubleday.

He, W. (2002). U.S. Census Bureau, Current Population Reports, Series P23-211, *The older foreign-born population of the United States, 2000*. U.S. Government Printing Office, Washington, DC.

Ho, D. (1986). Chinese patterns of socialization. In M. Bond (Ed.), *The psychology of the Chinese people* (pp. 1-37). Hong Kong: Oxford University Press.

Ho, D.Y.F. (1996). Filial piety and its psychological consequences. In M.H. Bond (Ed.), *The handbook of Chinese psychology*. Hong Kong: Oxford University Press.

Homans, G.C. (1958). Social behavior as exchange. *American Journal of Sociology*, 42, 597-606.

Hon, T-K. (1996). Ethnic and cultural pluralism: Gu Jiegang's vision of a new China in his studies of ancient history. *Modern China*, 22, 315-339.

Ivey, A. E., Ivey, M.B., & Simek-Morgan, L. (1997). *Counseling and psychotherapy: A multicultural perspective*. Boston: Allyn & Bacon.

Lee, M.Y., & Mjelde-Mossey, L.A. (in press). Cultural dissonance among generations: A solution-focused approach with East Asian elders and their families. *Journal of Marital & Family Therapy*.

Li, W.G. (2002). The cultural interaction between fashion and customs: The folk customs analysis of the grand triangle structure of Chinese culture among Beijing, Shanghai, and Henan. *Journal of An Yang Normal University*, 86, 70-71.

Liang, J., Krause, N.M., & Bennet, J.M. (2001). Social exchange and well-being: Is giving better than receiving? *Psychology and Aging*, 16, 511-523.

Mok, M.E. (2001). Empowerment of cancer patients from a Chinese perspective. *Nursing Ethics*, 8, 69-76.

Pijls, L.T.J., Feskens, E.J.M., & Kromhout, D. (1993). Self-rated health, mortality, and chronic disease in elderly men. *American Journal of Epidemiology*, 138, 840-848.

Pu, S.X., Chen, D.Y., & Zhou, Y. (1995). *An introduction to administrative divisions in Peoples Republic of China*. Beijing: Zhishi Publishing House (Chinese).

SPSS, Inc. (1999). *Statistical Package for the Social Sciences, 9.0*. Chicago, IL: Author.

Stryker, S. (1980). *Symbolic interactionism: A Social structural version*. Menlo Park, CA: Benjamin Cummings.

Sue, D.W. (1981). Dimensions of worldviews: Cultural identity. In *Issues and concepts in Cross-cultural counseling*. New York: John Wiley & Sons.

Sue, D.W., Ivey, A.E., & Pedersen, P.B. (1996). *A theory of multicultural counseling and therapy*. Pacific Grove, CA: Brooks/Cole.

Thibaut, J.W., & Kelley, H.H. (1959). *The social psychology of groups*. New York: Wiley.

Walster, E., Walster, G.W., & Berscheid, E. (1978). *Equity theory and research*. Boston: Allyn & Bacon.

Wu, H. (2002). Perceived talent from job advertisement: A comparison between Beijing, Shanghai, and Guangzhou. *China Talent*, 11, 14-16.

Xiangqun, C. (1999). Fat pigs and women's gifts: Agnatic and non-agnatic social support in Kaixiangong village. In J. West, Z. Minghua, C. Xiangqun, & C. Yuan (Eds.), *Women of China: Economic and social transformation*. New York: St. Martin's Press.

Xie, B. Zhao, X.H., Jia, J.B., Wu, Q.L., Su, Y.X., Chen, X.S., & Chen, C.M. (1997). Survey on nutritional knowledge, attitude, and practice among the residents in Beijing, Guangzhou, and Shanghai. *Journal of Hygiene Research*, 26, 343-348.

Yang, K.S. (1995). Chinese social orientation: An integrative analysis. In T.Y. Lin, W.S. Tseng, & E.K. Yeh (Eds.), *Chinese societies and mental health* (pp. 19-39). Hong Kong: Oxford University Press.

Zhang, S. (2002). Urban transformation: Remarks on reading Beijing, Shanghai, and Guangzhou. *Time Architecture*, 3, 34-37.

Zhang, J., & Bond, M.H. (1998). Personality and filial piety among college students in two Chinese societies: The added value of indigenous constructs. *Journal of Cross-Cultural Psychology*, 29, 402-416.

Zhao, X.H. Xie, B., Lin, Y., Su, Y.X., Wu, Q.L., & Chen, C.M. (1998). Survey on breakfast eating behavior among residents in Beijing, Guangzhou, and Shanghai. *Journal of Hygiene Research*, 27, 273-275.

The Rap Music Attitude
and Perception (RAP) Scale:
Scale Development and Preliminary Analysis
of Psychometric Properties

Edgar H. Tyson

SUMMARY. Rap music has become a vital part of youth culture and, consequently, is now a central component in many programs that serve youth. Understanding attitudes towards and perceptions of rap music can be an important step in informing various approaches to incorporating rap music into programs aimed at youth. This article reports the initial psychometric properties of the RAP. The RAP is an instrument designed to measure attitudes towards and perceptions of rap music. A review of the research on rap music revealed that although several re-

Edgar H. Tyson, PhD, MSW, is affiliated with the Florida State University, School of Social Work, C 2527 University Center, Tallahassee, FL 32306-2570 (E-mail: etyson@ mailer.fsu.edu).

This paper was supported in part by a CSWE/SAMHSA Doctoral Fellowship in Clinical Training awarded to the author.

The author thanks John Lounsbury and John Orme for assistance with the data analyses for this project. The author also thanks the blind reviewers for their helpful comments. A special thanks is extended to the students who volunteered to provide the data for this study and the youths who continue to inspire work contained in this paper.

[Haworth co-indexing entry note]: "The Rap Music Attitude and Perception (RAP) Scale: Scale Development and Preliminary Analysis of Psychometric Properties." Tyson, Edgar H. Co-published simultaneously in *Journal of Human Behavior in the Social Environment* (The Haworth Social Work Practice Press, an imprint of The Haworth Press, Inc.) Vol. 11, No. 3/4, 2005, pp. 59-82; and: *Approaches to Measuring Human Behavior in the Social Environment* (ed: William R. Nugent) The Haworth Social Work Practice Press, an imprint of The Haworth Press, Inc., 2005, pp. 59-82. Single or multiple copies of this article are available for a fee from The Haworth Document Delivery Service [1-800-HAWORTH, 9:00 a.m. - 5:00 p.m. (EST). E-mail address: docdelivery@haworthpress.com].

59

searchers discuss and interpret rap music attitudes and perceptions, a reliable and valid measure of these constructs is absent from the literature. Findings support a three-factor model of the RAP. Scale items loaded on their respective factors ranging from .55 to .83 and reliability analyses determined that the RAP and its three subscales had good internal consistency (i.e., α ranged from .87 to .92). Criterion validity results were also presented. Practical applications and future research of the RAP in social work practice with youth, their families and their communities were discussed. *[Article copies available for a fee from The Haworth Document Delivery Service: 1-800-HAWORTH. E-mail address: <docdelivery@haworthpress.com> Website: <http://www.HaworthPress.com> © 2005 by The Haworth Press, Inc. All rights reserved.]*

KEYWORDS. Hip hop, rap music, attitudes and perceptions, cultural assessment of youth

INTRODUCTION

The study of contributions of rap music is an important issue because it may be a highly effective tool to communicate with adolescents and young adults (Elligan, 2004; Tyson, 2003; Stokes & Gant, 2002). Although rap music has become the most popular music among adolescents and young adults in the United States and throughout the world (Farley, 1999), we know little about attitudes and perceptions people have towards this controversial art form. The increased significance in popular culture has led to a growing body of both conceptual and empirical research on rap music (Dixon & Brooks, 2002; Dixon & Linz, 1997; Lewis, Thompson, Celious, & Brown, 2002; Tyson, 2002). Negative attitudes and perceptions of rap music also appear to have received considerable attention in empirical research (Dixon & Brooks, 2002; Lewis et al., 2002; Lynxwiler & Gay, 2000; Tyson, 2002). Despite these criticisms of rap music, there have been limited reports (e.g., Kuwahara, 1992) with a specific focus of assessing positive attitudes towards rap music. More important, rigorous studies that have systematically investigated overall attitudes and perceptions of rap music are absent from the literature. A consequence of this gap in research is that a reliable and valid scale that measures attitudes and perceptions of rap music does not exist. Therefore, the development of a measure that assesses constructs of rap music attitudes and perceptions would be a significant contribution to the growing body of research on rap music.

Why Create a Measure for Rap Music Attitudes and Perceptions?

Understanding Youth Social and Cultural Environment. The development of an assessment tool that measures rap music attitudes and perceptions is relevant to understanding the social and cultural environment of our youth, particularly African American and Latino youth. Rap music is embedded in a larger youth culture called the "Hip Hop Culture," which for a large portion of the youth that social workers currently serve is a way of life and a way of viewing and interacting with the world (Rose, 1994; Stokes & Gant, 2002). Hip hop movies, plays, books, and clothing are pervasive in the commercial enterprise of mainstream American society. Because of the influence of hip hop, rap music is one of the most relevant and vital aspects of youth culture today, and a complete understanding and awareness of the behavior of youth include understanding youth culture. Arguably, there is no single more important influence on youth culture than hip hop and rap music, leading some scholars to advocate that in order for helping professionals to move toward "youth cultural competence" they must become aware of, sensitive to, and knowledgeable about the "Hip Hop Culture" (De Jesus, 2003; Elligan, 2004).

Developing an understanding of the culture of various client populations has been one of the primary components of the human behavior in social environment perspective (Longress, 2000; Zastrow & Kirst-Ashman, 1994). One view of the social environment is that it is an interaction between micro-systems and macro-systems, and culture is a vital part of the macro-system (Zastrow & Kirst-Ashman, 1994). Developing a working understanding of the cultural values and practices that drive and shape rap music and that are expressed through rap music might be particularly useful to social workers in their attempts to find ways to intervene with youth and young adults. More important, the development of a reliable and valid assessment tool to measure attitudes and perceptions of rap music might be an important first step in helping practitioners to gain more knowledge on what has become one of the most popular and influential cultural phenomena of the new millennium.

Screening Youth for Programs Incorporating Rap Music. Few would disagree that rap music is a central aspect of the culture of many youth in general and African American youth in particular. The importance of rap music to youth has given rise to the development of innovative approaches to integrating rap music in youth programs. For example, De Jesus (2003) recently conducted extensive, qualitative interviews of program directors and direct care staff from 10 of what are considered "groundbreaking" youth programs around the country utilizing hip hop and rap music to transform the lives of youth. One outreach program evaluated by De Jesus is "Friends of Island Academy" in New York City. This program uses rap music to engage, recruit and empower youth who are in the juvenile justice system and are preparing to make the transition from incarceration back into their neighborhoods (De Jesus, 2003). This program has an *"Art Group"* component that helps youth learn to channel their emotions through self-expression and exploration using poetry and music. The Maya Angelou Charter School, a similar program in Washington, DC, offers academic/career development, work experience and support services to ex-juvenile offenders. At Maya Angelou, youth achieve rigorous learning goals and critical thinking skills through the use of music (rap), writing (poetry), and other artistic mediums.

A final example of an innovative youth program that incorporates rap music is the "Hip Hop Center" at the University of Pennsylvania (De Jesus, 2003). Located in downtown Philadelphia, the center's two primary initiatives are: (1) the *African American Language and Culture Project*–an after-school program for 1st through 4th graders that uses rhyme and cultural themes to motivate students to make reading fun, and (2) the *Media Project*–a course for high school students, which includes an analysis of hip hop music and culture. An interesting component of the Hip Hop Center is that it trains youth in computer, video, and multimedia skills which facilitates its own research projects geared towards analyzing various aspects of Philadelphia's hip hop scene. The rationale for this study is that a tool that measures rap music attitudes and perceptions can be helpful in screening youth who might need to examine and change their endorsement of the negative aspects of rap music before becoming involved in interventions that have rap music as a core component.

CONSTRUCTS IN THE LITERATURE ON RAP MUSIC

The specific items included in the RAP were created to reflect the various constructs of rap music attitudes and perceptions found in the literature. After an exhaustive review of the literature there were three constructs of RAP music that became apparent. Although there were a number of different descriptions and representations of these constructs, there were strong and consistent similarities that tied the descriptions together to form each of the three constructs. The three constructs that were consistently represented in the literature were, "violent-misogynistic," "empowerment/positive," and "artistic-esthetic" attitudes towards and perceptions of rap music. Below is an in-depth discussion of what lead to the expectation that attitudes towards rap music would be expressed by way of these three general domains.

Violent-Misogynistic Construct

From the limited reviews of the literature that do exist, there appears to be two general attitudes towards rap music, one that is primarily negative and the other primarily positive (Dixon & Brooks, 2002; Thompson & Brown, 2002; Tyson, 2003). Dixon and Brooks (2002) examined some of the literature on rap music and found that early interest was mainly in rap as a cultural expression, and more recent attention has been an alarmist response to the misogynous and violent themes in rap music. Rap as violent has unfortunately been among the most popular constructs of rap music (Binder, 1993; Fenster, 1995). In the empirical literature (e.g., Barongan & Hall, 1995; Johnson, Jackson, & Gatto, 1995), it appears that most of the research has focused on the effects of violent, sexist and misogynous rap music (Thompson & Brown, 2002; Tyson, in press). Therefore, it is expected that a "violent-misogynistic" factor will be present when measuring attitudes toward rap music. This factor represents the perception that the content (i.e., lyrics) and culture of rap music primarily reflect violent, sexist, and misogynistic images. Although violent and sexist constructs have dominated the literature, there are positive constructs of rap as well.

Empowerment Construct

For more than a decade, several scholars and practitioners in the field of adolescent mental health and education have studied the potential of rap music to be used as a positive influence with youth (Cella, Tulsky, Sarafian, Thomas, & Thomas, 1992; De Carlo, 2000; Tyson, 2002, 2004; Stokes & Gant, 2002; Watts, Abdul-Adil, & Pratt, 2002). Cella et al. (1992) reported that an innovative smoking prevention program that included the use of rap music was successful with a group of elementary school children. More recently, research on innovative, therapeutic applications of rap music in group-work with adolescents has been published in the literature (De Carlo, 2000; Tyson, in press; Watts et al., 2002). A common theme in recent research is that there is theoretical support and empirical evidence for rap music's "empowering" qualities. For example, Watts et al. (2002) described a psycho-educational program called the *Young Warriors* that uses rap music to develop a "critical consciousness" in its young participants to help them deal with their daily struggles. Another example is Elligan's (2004) "rap therapy" model, where he uses case studies to describe how to assess a young person's interest in rap music, develop an individualized plan and conduct meaningful, purposeful counseling incorporating rap music. Moreover, in a compelling analysis on rap music, Rose (1994) concluded that rap music has made a significant impact on critical-consciousness and resistance to oppressive conditions. It must be noted that "critical-conscious raising" is one of the major components of the empowerment model of social work practice (Lee, 1994).

There is some empirical evidence to support the theory that rap music portrays an image of resistance to oppressive conditions (Kuwahara, 1992). Kuwahara summarized that, "rap music gives [African Americans] a feeling of power, and there is pleasure in feeling power and resisting the forces of domination" (p. 68). While Kuwahara's study had methodological limitations and has not yet been replicated, it offers preliminary evidence that suggests rap music has certain "empowering" qualities. Furthermore, Tyson (2002, 2003) provided evidence for and practical applications of a rap music intervention in social work practice with youth that is fundamentally linked to the intrinsic motivation and self-efficacy this type of intervention engenders in youth. Therefore, a second construct that is expected to emerge when measuring attitudes towards rap music is "empowerment," which represents the notion that rap music critiques oppressive conditions in the social environment and motivates young people to better understand how to counteract those conditions.

Artistic-Esthetic Construct

Although the majority of rap music research has documented a negative, destructive construct, and to a lesser extent, a positive, empowerment construct, there are likely to be many people who listen to rap music for its artistic and esthetic value. Since its inception, rap music was created out of a sense of enjoyment and was (and likely still is) primarily used to enhance the dance party (Rose, 1994). While some might disagree, rap music is by definition "music" and fundamentally has entertainment value. This aspect of rap music appears to have been lost in the controversy and debate surrounding some of its content. It is abundantly clear that several scholars agree that rap music represents a valid form of artistic expression rooted in the African American culture and tradition (Dixon & Linz, 1997; Dyson, 1995; Rose, 1994).

There is some limited empirical support for an artistic construct in rap music attitudes (Kuwahara, 1992). Kuwahara surveyed a sample of Caucasian American and African American students from two separate college campuses and reported that both groups endorsed rap music more for its artistic qualities, than for any other reason. Although there were several differences between the two groups of students, when asked why they listened to rap music, both groups of students overwhelmingly responded that they appreciated rap music for its beats and dance-related qualities. Therefore, a third factor that might emerge from an empirical examination of rap music attitude and perception constructs can be described as an "artistic-esthetic factor."

Purpose of the Study and Specific Hypotheses Tested

In moving towards a better understanding of how rap music impacts important social problems such as youth at-risk for behavior problems, it seems that a logical step in the advancement of knowledge in this area would be to develop a standard measure that assesses rap music attitudes and perceptions. The Rap Music Attitude and Perception (RAP) scale was developed as a measure of three constructs related to rap music. These constructs represent the three RAP subscales, which are Violent-Misogynistic (VM), Empowerment (EMP), and Artistic-Esthetic (AE). This study is the first known attempt to develop and validate a scale that measures specific constructs related to perceptions of and attitudes towards rap music. Specifically, the purpose of this study was to: (1) evaluate the reliability, factor validity, and criterion validity of the RAP scale; and (2) examine ethnic, gender, and age effects in total and subscale scores on the RAP.

It was hypothesized that the exploratory factor analyses will support the theoretical three-factor model of the RAP. A second hypothesis, that the RAP will have good reliability and validity, was also tested in this study. Specifically, in terms of validity, it was expected that rap music purchasing and listening habits will be positively associated with RAP total and subscale scores, and support of censorship of rap music will be negatively associated with RAP total and subscale scores. These criteria used to validate the RAP were selected because of their practical significance and previous research. Intuitively, it is likely that owning rap music CDs and tapes, as well as listening to rap music, are indications that a person has a more positive attitude toward and perception of rap music. More specifically, it is unlikely that a person would spend their valuable dollars purchasing a product that they prefer not to listen to. It is equally unlikely that a person would spend their valuable time listening to music that they do not enjoy. In terms of censorship of rap music, previous research suggests that favoring censorship of rap music is likely to indicate that a person has a more negative perception of the music genre (Lynxwiler & Gay, 2000). The rationale here is that few people would favor the censorship of a music format that they perceived as being generally positive.

METHOD

Identification of RAP Items

Twenty-six items were identified to assess rap music attitudes and perceptions. Because no existing scale that measures attitudes towards rap music was found in the literature, a novel approach to item development was undertaken in this pilot study. After reviewing the literature, 110 items were written that described the most common views, statements and attitudes that consistently appeared in the literature. Based on common themes, this initial pool of 110 items was narrowed to 26. To determine their face validity, the list of 26 items was given to four colleagues and four young adults who were known to have a personal appreciation for rap music. After a few minor adjustments, all eight reviewers endorsed the revised list of 26 items. The 26 items of the RAP scale are presented in Table 1.

Scale Format. Each item was presented in a 5-point Likert-scale format (1 = Strongly Disagree, 2 = Disagree, 3 = Neutral, 4 = Agree, 5 = Strongly Agree). There were twelve negatively worded items that were reversed coded (see Table 1) in order for higher scores on the total scale and its three subscales to indicate more positive attitudes. Thus, total scale scores and subscale scores were calculated using the summed scores of the corresponding items. Range in scores on the final RAP scale and its subscales, along with final items for each subscale, are presented in the results.

TABLE 1. Initial RAP Items

1. Rap music expresses legitimate frustration with social conditions.
2. Rap music has positive themes that uplift and empower people.
3. Some rap music teaches youth how to make it through bad times.
4. Youth relate to rap music because it is about their reality.
5. Some rap music represents a form of resistance to oppressive conditions.
6. *Sexually explicit rap music causes males to be sexually explicit with females.
7. *Violent rap music videos can lead males to be more violent.
8. Rap music is a progression of African and African American storytelling.
9. There are very important messages in rap.
10. *Rap music expresses negative attitudes towards homosexuality.
11. *Most rap music suggests women are *just* for male sexual satisfaction.
12. I like rap music for its beats and use of sound.
13. I like rap music for its content and its messages.
14. *All gansta rap music has negative messages.
15. *Rap music is not a real form of music, it's just talking over sounds.
16. *Rappers are not really as talented musicians as most other musicians.
17. Rappers have a creative form of intelligence.
18. *Competition between rappers is dangerous and leads to violence.
19. *Rap music projects macho attitudes.
20. Rap music helps youth cope with their reality.
21. Rap music encourages ethnic group pride.
22. Rap music is a healthy resistance against the system.
23. *Violence in rap videos contributes to aggressive behaviors.
24. *Sexism in rap videos contributes to sexist behaviors.
25. *Rap music glorifies drugs and violence.
26. Rap reflects the realities of drugs and violence in society.

*Items were reverse coded.

Design

A correlational design was used to conduct this study. The RAP was pilot tested using a nonrandom sample of college students from a predominantly white institution in the southeastern United States during the Fall semester, 2002. Most of the students were enrolled in an Introductory Psychology, Social Work Policy, or Social Work and Oppression course. Some students were members of a student organization.[1]

Data Collection and Sample Characteristics

The RAP scale was administered to students in their classrooms or organizational meeting. A total of 275 surveys was distributed. There were 248 students who completed and returned the surveys. The 248 respondents represent a 90.2% response rate. Although no information was obtained on the 9.8% non-responders, there was no evidence to suggest that these 27 students were systematically different from the students who responded to the surveys. The ages of the participants ranged from 19 years to 53 years ($M = 26.0$ years, $SD = 7.2$), and approximately 167 were female and 78 were male. Caucasian Americans made up 64% (n = 160) and African Americans comprised 31.8% (n = 78) of the sample. Complete participant demographics are reported in Table 2.

Finally, there were several criterion-related validity questions that were included in the surveys. Specifically, participants were asked to report: (1) the number of rap music CDs or tapes owned; (2) how often they listened to rap music; and (3) whether or not they favored more censorship of rap music.

Data Analyses

Reliability and validity analyses were conducted on the RAP scale. For factor validity analysis, a "restricted" form of Exploratory Factor Analysis (EFA) was conducted using the Principal Component Analysis (PCA) extraction method to test whether these data would support

TABLE 2. Participant Demographics (N = 248)

Age[a]:	$M = 26.0$ years	$SD = 7.2$ years	Range = 19-53 years
Gender:	Female	67.3%	(n = 167)
	Male	31.5%	(n = 78)
	Missing	1.2%	(n = 3)
Ethnicity:	Caucasian American	64.5%	(n = 160)
	African American	31.5%	(n = 78)
	Hispanic	1.2%	(n = 3)
	Asian-Pacific Islander	.8%	(n = 2)
	Jamaican-American	.4%	(n = 1)
	American-Indian	.4%	(n = 1)
	Missing	1.2%	(n = 3)

[a]Eight participants did not report age.

the hypothesized three-factor model of the RAP. This method is referred to as "restricted" factor analysis (Anderson & Gerbing, 1988) because a set number of factors (i.e., three) that are expected to represent the data were specified, adding a constraint on the data. To justify this approach, an initial and strictly EFA procedure was used to first assess the number of factors that would result using the "initial eigenvalue greater than one" rule. As expected, three factors fell from the data during this initial phase. As shown in Table 3, the EMP factor accounted for 37.25% of the variance in the model. The VM factor accounted for an additional 11.57% of the variance and the AE factor accounted for 8.92% of the variance in the model. Therefore, 57.79% of the total variance in rap music attitudes and perceptions was explained by the three-factor model.

Some might argue that EFA is not appropriate when the underlying constructs are well-defined (Fabrigar, Wegener, MacCallum, & Strahan, 1999), as is the case with the RAP. However, this is the initial test of the RAP model and no other scale that validates these constructs exists. To address these somewhat opposing views, a "restricted" EFA approach of setting the number of rotated factors in the model at "three" was determined to be the most appropriate approach to the factor analysis in this study (Anderson & Gerbing, 1988). This procedure remained exploratory because each item was free to load on a specified number of factors. The restricted EFA approach was a reasonable compromise because it added a constraint to the data, while maintaining a necessary level of exploratory freedom in the model. Finally, in these analyses, an oblique rotation was used because it assumes the factors are correlated, which is usually the case (Fabrigar et al., 1999).

After conducting the factor analysis of the RAP, reliability analyses were conducted. For reliability, coefficient alphas were analyzed for the total scale and each subscale. For criterion-related validity analyses, bivariate correlations between RAP total and subscale scores and crite-

TABLE 3. Initial Exploratory Factor Analysis Results

Factor	Eigenvalue	% of Variance	Cum. Var.	Label
1	9.68	37.25	37.25	Empowerment
2	2.99	11.57	48.82	Violent-Misogynistic
3	1.87	8.97	57.79	Artistic-Esthetic

rion variables were conducted. Because the RAP includes subscales, intercorrelations of the scale and subscales were conducted and presented. Additional bivariate correlations were conducted between RAP scores, criterion variables and demographic data. Although not specifically hypothesized, it was expected that being young, African American, and male would be positively correlated with RAP scores.

Caveat of Performing Multiple Significance Tests

An important caveat must be noted regarding the number of correlations that were performed in this study. With an increase in the number of significance tests, the probability of making Type I errors (i.e., rejection of the null hypothesis when it is, in fact, true) increases at a corresponding rate (Cohen & Cohen, 1983). A common solution to the Type I error problem is to make a correction, such as the Bonferroni correction, to the overall alpha level. The Bonferroni test includes dividing the overall alpha level (typically $p = .05$) by the number of significance tests being performed and setting the alpha level of each test at the resulting p value. Unfortunately, this minimizes the risk of Type I errors at the expense of a substantial reduction in power, thus making Type II errors (failure to reject the null hypothesis when the null is, in fact, false) more likely. While there are no hard or fast rules for making decisions regarding these matters, for the purposes of this exploratory study, with each set of statistical tests performed, the overall alpha level was set at $p = .10$ in order to minimize the reduction in power (i.e., probability of avoiding Type II errors). For each set of statistical tests, the p value applied to each individual test after making the Bonferroni correction is noted where appropriate.

RESULTS

Factor Analytic Structure of the RAP

EFA was conducted, specifying that three factors would represent these data well. As expected, the three-factor model of the RAP was supported by the EFA results, which are shown in Table 4. Specifically, the loading of each item appears consistent with the appropriate hypothesized construct. Loadings, also called parameter estimates, are the correlations between the original variables or items and the factors. The factor loadings on factor 1, the EMP factor, ranged from .487 to .784.

TABLE 4. Factor Loadings[a] of the RAP (N = 248)

Item	Factor		
	Empowerment	Violent-Misogynistic	Artistic-Esthetic
20	.791	.157	−.002
2	.742	.298	.005
3	.741	.175	.212
9	.695	.002	.271
4	.694	.120	−.002
21	.680	.009	.137
22	.635	.195	.255
5	.607	−.002	.299
1	.607	−.007	.300
13	.572	.304	.323
8	.567	.157	.218
24	.131	.834	.106
23	.009	.814	.229
7	.140	.753	.230
6	.170	.746	.111
18	.006	.654	.219
25	.313	.649	.004
11	.412	.635	.191
19	.005	.610	.001
10	.002	.606	.007
15	.182	.290	.776
17	.370	.001	.732
16	.254	.308	.701
12	.160	.115	.681
14*	.194	.375	.537

[a]Set number of factors at three. Extraction method: Principal Component Analysis. Rotation method: Oblique.
*Because of a poor loading pattern, this item was discarded from the scale and not part of subsequent analyses.

As shown in Table 4, these items did not load above .3 on the other two factors suggesting that they diverged appropriately from the other factors of the RAP scale.

Similar to the EMP factor, all but one of the items that were expected to load on the VM factor were high, ranging from .606 to .834. Item 14 presented a problem because it loaded .375 on the VM factor. Using a conservative standard for parameter estimates (i.e., ≥ .400), item 14 did not appear to load well on the VM factor (Loehlin, 1988). Additionally, there was a problem with item 14 because it loaded .537 on the AE factor. Because theoretically, it did not make sense to add this item to the AE factor, item 14 was discarded and was not part of subsequent analyses. This resulted in a VM factor that had 9 items. All but one of these 9 items did not load well (i.e., above .400) on the other two factors. Item 11 loaded .412 on the EMP factor and might represent reason for caution in using this item to identify a VM construct. However, it has been suggested that differences in parameter estimates below .2 are not as problematic when differentiating between constructs (Loehlin, 1988). Therefore, because item 11 loaded .635 on the VM factor and represents a difference greater than .2 from the .412 loading on the AE factor, this item was retained.

The third and final construct was also supported by these data. There were four initial AE items and all were retained because their loadings on the AE factor were high, ranging from .681 to .776. These four items also diverged well from the EMP and VM factors. Therefore, it appears that the theoretical three-factor model of the RAP scale was represented by these data.

Reliability of Final RAP and Subscales

Total and subscale mean scores and reliabilities of the RAP are presented in Table 5. The final RAP scale consisted of 25 items, and its alpha suggests it has good internal consistency (i.e., α = .92). Possible total scores on the RAP range from 25 to 125 and higher scores represent more positive attitudes and perceptions of rap music. The mean

TABLE 5. RAP Mean Scores, Standard Deviations (SD), Standard Errors (SE), and Alpha Reliabilities (N = 248)

Scale	Mean *(SD)*	*S.E.*	Internal Consistency
RAP	81.38 (14.75)	1.01	α = .92
Empowerment	41.33 (9.12)	.56	α = .90
Violent-Misogynistic	24.58 (6.70)	.46	α = .89
Artistic-Esthetic	15.92 (3.23)	.22	α = .87

score of this sample was 81.38 (*SD* = 14.75). This mean appears to suggest that the present sample had relatively mixed (i.e., positive and negative), although somewhat more positive rather than negative, attitudes and perceptions of rap music. The EMP subscale consisted of 12 items and possible scores range from 12 to 60. The alpha for the EMP subscale was α = .90, suggesting that it has good internal consistency. The mean EMP score of this sample was 41.33 (*SD* = 9.12). This high mean suggests that the present sample had a relatively high EMP attitude and perception toward rap music. The VM subscale consisted of 9 items and possible scores range from 9 to 45, with higher scores representing more positive VM attitudes. The alpha for this subscale was α = .89. The mean VM score for this sample was 24.58 (*SD* = 6.70) suggesting that this sample did not endorse the view that rap music is mostly violent, sexist and misogynistic. Finally, the AE subscale consisted of four items and possible scores range from 4 to 20. The reliability of the AE factor was also good (i.e., α = .87). The mean AE score for this sample was 15.92 (*SD* = 3.23). This high score suggests that on average the present sample endorsed the view that rap music does have artistic and esthetic value. The results of the EFA and the reliability analyses partially support the hypothesis that the RAP will have good psychometric properties.

Criterion Validity Analyses

The criterion validity analyses were conducted by generating validity coefficients for the RAP and each of its three subscales (see Table 6). These validity coefficients were interpreted using Cohen's (1992) standard for effect sizes (i.e., small = .1, moderate = .3, and large = .5). The Bonferroni correction made to the set of 12 statistical tests performed

TABLE 6. Criterion Validities of the RAP

Criterion	Scale			
	RAP	EMP	VM	AE
Listen to rap (n = 247)	.40**	.39**	.19**	.35**
Own rap music (n = 248)	.45**	.46**	.23**	.24**
Favor censorship (n = 247)	−.51**	−.52**	−.18**	−.36**

**p < .008 (2-tailed)

here, suggested that the alpha level applied to each individual test should be set at $p = .008$.

The RAP total scores were moderately associated with rap music-listening habits. As expected, higher scores on the RAP scale were positively correlated with the amount of time spent listening to rap music (i.e., $r = .40, p < .008$). Also as expected, the RAP was moderately associated with whether or not participants owned rap music (i.e., $r = .45, p < .008$) and had a large association with whether or not they favored censorship of rap music (i.e., $r = -.51, p < .008$). These results suggest that the RAP scale had good criterion validity because it was significantly associated with the criteria used in this study in the direction predicted and the effect sizes of these associations were in the moderate to large range.

The subscales of the RAP also appear to have good criterion validity. Higher EMP scores were positively correlated with the amount of time spent listening to rap music (i.e., $r = .39, p < .008$). EMP scores were also moderately correlated, in the direction predicted, with whether or not participants owned rap music (i.e., $r = .46, p < .008$). Finally, as expected, higher EMP scores had a large, negative correlation with the extent to which participants favored censorship of rap music (i.e., $r = -.52, p < .008$). These results suggest that the EMP subscale was significantly associated with the criteria used in this study in the direction predicted and the effect sizes of these associations were in the moderate to large range.

Higher (i.e., more positive) VM scores had a small, positive correlation with the amount of time spent listening to rap music (i.e., $r = .19, p < .008$). VM scores also had a small association in the predicted direction with whether or not participants owned rap music (i.e., $r = .23, p < .008$), and a small, negative correlation with the extent to which participants favored censorship of rap music (i.e., $r = -.18, p < .008$). These validity coefficients, although small, were in the direction predicted and suggest that the VM subscale had fairly good criterion validity.

Finally, higher (i.e., more positive) AE scores had a moderate, positive correlation with the amount of time spent listening to rap music (i.e., $r = .35, p < .008$) and a small, positive association with whether or not participants owned rap music (i.e., $r = .24, p < .008$). As expected, AE scores were negatively correlated with the extent to which participants favored censorship of rap music (i.e., $r = -.36, p < .008$). These validity coefficients were in the small-to-moderate range and suggest that the AE subscale had good criterion validity. The criterion-validity results appear to be consistent with the hypothesis the RAP and its subscales will have good psychometric properties.

Intercorrelations

The intercorrelations of the RAP are presented in Table 7. Because of the low number of tests (i.e., six) and the substantially high probability of statistical significance of all intercorrelations (i.e., scores from the RAP and its subscales are highly likely to be related), no Bonferroni correction was made. Overall, these results show that the RAP subscales are moderately correlated with each other and strongly correlated with the full RAP scale. With the exception of the correlation between the AE and EMP subscales (i.e., $r = .54$, $p < .001$), all intercorrelations met the standard for moderate effect size as determined by Cohen (1992). The strong effect size of .54 appears to suggest that the overlap in variance of overall rap music attitudes and perceptions between the AE and EMP factors might be greater than expected. Nonetheless, taken together, the intercorrelations and the EFA results appear to confirm that the three constructs represent sufficiently different aspects of overall rap music attitudes and perceptions. A comprehensive examination of the results of this initial analysis of the RAP seems to suggest that it has good psychometric properties.

Bivariate Correlations of Demographic Data

The results of the bivariate correlations between demographic variables and RAP total and subscale scores, as well as criterion questions, were mixed and are presented in Table 8. The Bonferroni correction

TABLE 7. Intercorrelations of the RAP

Scale	Scale			
	RAP	EMP	VM	AE
RAP	-	.86***	.78***	.73***
EMP		-	.42***	.54***
VM			-	.45***
AE				-

***$p < .001$ (2-tailed)

TABLE 8. Bivariate Correlations Between RAP and Demographic Variables[a]

	Age (N = 240)	Gender (N = 241)	Ethnicity[b] (N = 244)
RAP	−.01	−.23**	−.30**
EMP	.07	−.25**	−.28**
VM	.11	−.19**	−.30**
AE	−.19**	−.02	−.20**

[a] Gender was coded male = 0, female = 1, and Ethnicity was coded African American = 0, Caucasian Americans = 1.
[b] Because there were so few subjects in the other ethnic groups represented in this study, and to simplify the statistical procedure, only African Americans and Caucasian Americans were included in these analyses.
**$p < .008$ (2-tailed)

made to the set of 12 statistical tests performed here, suggested that the alpha level applied to each individual test should be set at $p = .008$. Age was not linearly related to total RAP, EMP, or VM scores. However, age did have a linear relationship with AE scores in the direction expected (i.e., $r = −.19, p < .008$), suggesting that younger participants had more positive AE rap music attitudes and perceptions. Younger participants also appear to listen to rap music more than their older counterparts ($r = −.36, p < .008$). In terms of owning rap music or favoring censorship, age did not appear to matter. However, because the mean age was 26 years in this sample, the restriction of range in age might have influenced these results.

As expected, African American subjects (coded "0") had more positive total RAP scores ($r = −.30, p < .008$), EMP scores ($r = −.28, p < .008$), VM scores ($r = −.30, p < .008$) and AE scores ($r = −.20, p < .008$) than Caucasian American subjects (coded "1"). In this sample it appears that African Americans also listened to ($r = −.21, p < .008$) and owned ($r = −.37, p < .008$) more rap music than Caucasian Americans. However, it does not appear that ethnicity mattered in terms of favoring censorship of rap music.

Finally, there were significant associations between gender and the validity criterion used in this study. Specifically, females (coded "1") had less positive RAP scores ($r = −.23, p < .008$), EMP scores ($r = −.25, p < .008$) and VM scores ($r = −.19, p < .008$) than males (coded "0"). In contrast, it appears that gender was not significantly related to AE scores. Moreover, in this sample males owned ($r = −.30, p < .008$) more rap music than their female counterparts. However, males were more likely to favor censorship of rap music ($r = .32, p < .008$) than their female counterparts. These results, their implications and suggestions on how the RAP scale can be applied in practice and future research are discussed below.

DISCUSSION

Limitations of the Study

The above results must be interpreted within the context of methodological limitations of this pilot study of the RAP. The RAP was administered to a convenience (i.e., nonrandom) sample of college students and the results obtained here might not generalize to the larger population. It might be that certain characteristics of people who have not attended college would contribute to them having different attitudes and perceptions regarding rap music. For example, although no information on SES of this sample was obtained, it is not unlikely that a disproportionate number of college students come from more affluent communities and families. People from less advantaged communities might have different attitudes and perceptions of rap music than the sample used in this study. This is an issue that can be addressed in future research by including samples with diverse SES backgrounds.

A second potential limitation of this study is that the constructs identified to represent rap music attitudes and perceptions might not be inclusive of the diversity in views towards this popular and yet controversial art form. It is likely that additional constructs of attitudes and perceptions regarding rap music could be reliably measured and validated. Furthermore, there might be considerable disagreement on the definitions of one or more of the constructs that are measured in the RAP scale. For example, there is some disagreement on what exactly is "empowerment." Some suggest that empowerment has an inherent "behavioral" component that cannot be captured in a person's "perception" or "attitude." Therefore, a scale that does not measure behavioral aspects of individuals cannot fully measure empowerment. However, the current constructs in the literature on rap music attitudes and perceptions appear to be fairly represented in the RAP scale. Additionally, whether or not an attitude or perception labeled "empowerment" translates into actual behavior remains an empirical question and should be pursued in future research. Indeed, the preliminary results of the RAP scale appear to support using the RAP to compare specific views people have about rap music to their behavior.

Finally, another potential weakness of these preliminary results is that they are by definition exploratory. The EFA and criterion validity results shown here might not be replicated using a similar sample of college students or a sample of younger subjects. The EFA and the criterion validity results must be replicated in order to increase our confidence that the RAP and its subscales are valid measures of the constructs that they propose to represent. For example, it would be important to conduct confirmatory factor analysis (CFA) of the RAP with a new sample. New research on the RAP is underway that will address this issue directly. It is expected that this new program of research will test whether the three-factor model found here could be confirmed using more stringent factor analytic procedures such as CFA.

Implications and Directions for Future Research

Despite the limitations mentioned above, the results of this study appear to provide important information in the advancement of knowledge on rap music attitudes and perceptions. The primary objective of this study was to examine the initial psychometric properties of the RAP scale and its subscales. One implication of this study is that we now know that three of the constructs of rap music attitudes and perceptions most often cited in the literature can be reliably measured. The final 25-item version of the RAP was found to have good internal consistency as a global measure and as a measure of three different rap music attitude and perception constructs (i.e., Empowerment, Violent-Misogynistic, and Artistic-Esthetic). Another implication of these findings is that it has now been empirically shown that there are both positive and negative rap music attitudes and perceptions and these constructs are valid representations of the current views of this art form found in the literature. Because rap music is an important method of communicating these constructs to youth, a screening tool such as the RAP is necessary. Specifically, the use of a reliable and valid measure is the most appropriate method of assessing the relative importance of pre-existing rap music attitudes and perceptions, in terms of how these views might influence the effectiveness of a manipulation or intervention.

Furthermore, it is important that we now have additional empirical evidence to support the theory that rap music appears to have more salience in the lives of African Americans than it has for some other ethnic groups. African Americans were consistently more likely to endorse more positive overall rap music attitudes and perceptions, as well as specific constructs of rap music in a more positive direction. This notion has repeatedly been reported in the conceptual literature and to a lesser extent in the empirical literature (e.g., Kuwahara, 1992). While there might be several reasons to study the impact and importance of negative aspects of rap music in the larger community, these results imply that studying the positive effects of rap music on African Americans would be appropriate. Specifically, continued failure to examine positive effects and aspects of rap music in the African American community represents a significant gap in the literature. However, future research must attempt to disentangle ethnicity from rap music attitudes and perception in order to better understand specific mechanisms that might attribute for differences in this relationship.

Future research must also examine the reliability and validity of the RAP with younger samples. The mean age of this sample was 26 years and the correlation between ages and listening to rap music (i.e., $r = -.36$) suggests that younger participants in this sample appeared to enjoy rap music more than did older participants. Additionally, the relevance of rap music in youth culture warrants further analysis of the RAP using younger samples. It is likely that because of the importance and popularity of rap music among youth, the psychometric properties of the RAP would fare equally well among younger members of the population. Including younger participants in future validation studies of the RAP might reveal important age differences in rap music attitudes and perceptions.

CONCLUSION

The RAP can provide social workers and other practitioners with a valuable tool to use in working with youth and young adults, particularly those in the African American and Latino community. For example, information obtained from youth about their rap music attitudes and perceptions can facilitate discussions about how they perceive the relative importance and impact of drugs, crime, and explicit sexual messages in their lives and on the broader community in which they live. The RAP might work well as a screening tool to identify misconceptions about the impact of these negative forces on the lives of youth and young adults in certain communities. More important from a strengths perspective, the information obtained from the RAP can help facilitate increased community action and involvement in improving negative social conditions, such as crime, drug activity, and premature sexual activity. The Empowerment scale can be particularly useful in providing a tool to assess and screen youth for their potential for forming community action groups, as well as monitoring change in their empowerment activities.

There is some evidence that using rap music in social work practice can enhance motivation for treatment for youth at-risk for emotional and behavioral problems and can be used as an effective means to enhance the attainment of treatment goals (De Jesus, 2003; Elligan, 2004; Tyson, 2002; in press). De Jesus (2003) discusses the top 10 innovative programs in the country that include a substantial rap music component in their work with youth. Attempts to transport these types of programs to other venues offer ideal opportunities for further development and use of the RAP. One potential use for the RAP would be to assess the attitudes and perceptions of constituents who might have a stake in or some control over whether or not such programs and interventions get implemented in their community. The assessment results could then be used to inform efforts to change or appeal to attitudes and perceptions towards rap music that these potential stakeholders might have.

Because programs that incorporate rap music are intended to improve certain outcomes for youth, the RAP could be used as an outcome measure to evaluate the effect these types of programs have had on youths' perceptions of rap music. Furthermore, youth with certain types of pre-existing views of rap music might fair better or worse than those with very different views towards rap music. Future research involving rap music should first assess the type of attitudes and perceptions potential participants have prior to applying a manipulation or intervention. These assessment results could then be used to inform efforts to change or appeal to attitudes and perceptions youth have regarding rap music, in order to maximize the effects of an intervention. It is possible that a rap music intervention might not be as effective with youth or young adults who have low scores on the VM subscale because this might indicate that they have rap music attitudes and perceptions that indicate the endorsement of the violent-misogynistic rap music. Conversely, youth and young adults who have positive views of rap music might be more likely to benefit from therapeutic interventions that include the use of rap music. Furthermore, social workers and other practitioners can use the RAP to assess the compatibility of views of rap music between parents and children. It might be that parent-child dyads with positive scores on the RAP can benefit from a family intervention that incorporates some aspect of rap music.

In conclusion, despite the limitations of this study, the final version of the RAP developed here has vast potential for applications in social work practice, particularly in terms of increasing our understanding of youth behavior in their social environment. With information from the RAP, practitioners can empower families and communities to engage in discourse surrounding important social problems such as crime, drugs, poverty, and economic and social oppression. Social work has a rich tradition of employing empowerment and strengths-based approaches to engaging individuals and families in attempts to improve their conditions. Failure to utilize a resource as important as the RAP would represent another missed opportunity for social workers and other practitioners to have a more positive presence in the lives of a large of group of people who they encounter in their daily practice.

NOTE

1. To ensure maximum participation of African American students, permission was granted to survey members of two African American student organizations during their respective general body meetings.

REFERENCES

Anderson, J. C., & Gerbing, D. W. (1988). Structural equation modeling in practice: A review and recommended two-step approach. *Psychological Bulletin, 103*, 411-423.

Barongan, C., & Nagayama-Hall, G. C. (1995). The influence of misogynous rap music on sexual aggression. *Psychology of Women Quarterly, 19*, 195-207.

Binder, A. (1993). Constructing racial rhetoric: Media depictions of harm in heavy metal and rap music. *American Sociological Review, 58*, 753-767.

Cella, D. F., Tulsky, D. S., Sarafian, B., Thomas, C. R, Jr., & Thomas, C. R., Sr. (1992). Culturally relevant smoking prevention for minority youth. *Journal of School Health, 62*, 377-380.

Cohen, J. (1992). A power primer. *Psychological Bulletin, 112*, 155-159.

Cohen, J., & Cohen, P. (1983). *Applied multiple regression/correlation analysis for the behavioral sciences* (2nd ed.). Hillside, NJ: Erlbaum.

De Carlo, A. (2001). Rap therapy?: An innovative approach to group-work with urban adolescents. *Journal of Intergroup Relations, 28*, 40-48.

De Jesus, E. (2003). *Youth cultural competence.* Maryland: Youth Development and Research Fund.

Dixon, T. L., & Brooks, T. (2002). Rap music and rap audiences: Controversial themes, psychological effects and political resistance. *African American Research Perspectives, 8*, 106-116.

Dixon, T. L., & Linz, D. G. (1997). Obscenity law and sexually explicit rap music: Understanding the effects of sex, attitudes, and beliefs. *Journal of Applied Communication Research, 25*, 217-241.

Dyson, M. E. (1996). *Between God and gangsta rap: Bearing witness to black culture.* New York: Oxford University Press.

Elligan, D. (2004). *Rap therapy: A guide for communicating with youth and young adults through rap music.* New York, NY: Defina.

Epstein J. S., Pratto, D. J., & Skipper, J. K. (1990). Teenagers' behavioral problems and preferences for metal & rap music: A case study of a southern middle school. *Deviant Behavior, 11,* 381-394.

Fabrigar, L. R., Wegener, D. T., MacCallum, R. C., & Strahan, E. J. (1999). Evaluating the use of exploratory factor analysis in psychological research. *Psychological Methods, 4,* 272-299.

Farley, J. (1999, February 8). Hip hop nation. *Time,* 54-64.

Fenster, M. (1995). Understanding and incorporating rap: The articulation of alternative popular musical practices within dominant cultural practices and institutions. *Howard Journal of Communications, 5,* 223-244.

Johnson, J. J., Jackson, L. A., & Gatto, L. (1995). Violent attitudes and deferred academic aspirations: Deleterious effects of exposure to rap music. *Basic and Applied Social Psychology, 16,* 27-41.

Kuwahara, Y. (1992). Power to the people y'all: Rap music, resistance, and black college students. *Humanity and Society, 16,* 54-73.

Lee, J. A. B. (1994). *The empowerment approach to social work practice.* New York: Columbia University Press.

Lewis, R. L., Thompson, M. E., Celious, A. K., & Brown, R. K. (2002). Rap music, is it really all bad? Why hip hop scholarship is important. *African American Research Perspectives, 8,* 67-69.

Loehlin, J. C. (1998). *Latent variable models: An introduction to factor path and structural analysis.* New Jersey: LEA.

Longress, J. F. (2002). *Human behavior in the social environment* (3rd ed.). Itasca, IL: F.E. Peacock.

Lynxwiler, J., & Gay, D. (2000). Moral boundaries and deviant music: Public attitudes toward heavy metal and rap. *Deviant Behavior, 21,* 63-85.

Rose, T. (1994). *Black noise: Rap music and black culture in contemporary America.* Hanover, NH: Wesleyan University Press.

Stokes, C. E., & Gant, L. M. (2002). Turning the tables on the HIV/AIDS epidemic: Hip hop as a tool for reaching African American adolescent girls. *African American Research Perspectives, 8,* 70-81.

Tyson, E. H. (2002). Hip hop therapy: An exploratory study of a rap music intervention in group therapy with at-risk and delinquent youth. *Journal of Poetry Therapy, 15,* 131-144.

Tyson, E. H. (in press). Rap music in social work practice with African American and Latino youth: A conceptual model with practical applications. *Human Behavior in the Social Environment.*

Watts, R. J., Abdul-Adil, J. K., & Pratt, T. (2002). Enhancing critical consciousness in young African American men: A psychoeducational approach. *Psychology of Men and Masculinity, 3,* 41-50.

Zastrow, C., & Kirst-Ashman, K. K. (1994). *Understanding human behavior and the social environment* (3rd ed.). Chicago, IL: Nelson-Hall.

Assessment of Self-Esteem Among Individuals with Severe Mental Illness: Testing Two Dimensions of Self-Esteem Theory and Implications for Social Work Practice

Sang Kyoung Kahng

Carol Mowbray

SUMMARY. This study examines whether the factor structure of the Rosenberg Self-Esteem Scale consists of two dimensions (Owens, 1993), and whether the two dimensions are associated with different predictive factors and behavioral outcomes among individuals with severe mental illness who are served by community-based, psychosocial rehabilitation agencies. Confirmatory factor analyses of data from these indi-

Sang Kyoung Kahng, PhD, is Assistant Professor, Department of Social Welfare, College of Social Science, Seoul National University.

Carol Mowbray, PhD, is affiliated with School of Social Work, University of Michigan, Ann Arbor, MI.

Address correspondence to: Sang Kyoung Kahng, PhD, Department of Social Welfare, College of Social Science, Seoul National University, San 56-1, Sillim-Dong, Gwanak-Gu, Seoul, 151-742, Korea.

This research was funded by NIMH grant # 1 RO3 MH64317-01A1 to the first author.

[Haworth co-indexing entry note]: "Assessment of Self-Esteem Among Individuals with Severe Mental Illness: Testing Two Dimensions of Self-Esteem Theory and Implications for Social Work Practice." Kahng, Sang Kyoung, and Carol Mowbray. Co-published simultaneously in *Journal of Human Behavior in the Social Environment* (The Haworth Social Work Practice Press, an imprint of The Haworth Press, Inc.) Vol. 11, No. 3/4, 2005, pp. 83-104; and: *Approaches to Measuring Human Behavior in the Social Environment* (ed: William R. Nugent) The Haworth Social Work Practice Press, an imprint of The Haworth Press, Inc., 2005, pp. 83-104. Single or multiple copies of this article are available for a fee from The Haworth Document Delivery Service [1-800-HAWORTH, 9:00 a.m. - 5:00 p.m. (EST). E-mail address: docdelivery@haworthpress.com].

doi:10.1300/J137v11n03_05

viduals indicated that the traditional global self-esteem scale does reflect two dimensions–i.e., self-enhancement and self-deprecation. Bivariate and multivariate analyses revealed that factors associated with self-enhancement differ from factors associated with self-deprecation. These findings support the validity of two dimensions of self-esteem. Implications for social work practice and research are presented. *[Article copies available for a fee from The Haworth Document Delivery Service: 1-800-HAWORTH. E-mail address: <docdelivery@haworthpress.com> Website: <http://www.HaworthPress.com> © 2005 by The Haworth Press, Inc. All rights reserved.]*

KEYWORDS. Self-esteem, measurement, mental illness, psychosocial rehabilitation, social work practice

Rosenberg (1965) defined self-esteem as a positive or negative attitude toward the self. As certain attitudes toward an object frequently entail corresponding psychological, social, or behavioral responses to the object (Petty et al., 1997), a person's self-esteem is closely associated with his/her psychological, social, and behavioral outcomes. Individuals with high self-esteem tend to adapt better when they exper- ience major stressors because they have more efficient coping strategies (Carver, Scheier, & Weinstraub, 1989). Self-esteem plays a role as an effective defense against stressful consequences and can prevent negative health and mental health outcomes (Pearlin, 1987; Lazarus & Folkman, 1984). It is, therefore, important for individuals to maintain certain levels of self-esteem to successfully cope with stressors and to achieve optimum outcomes. Thus, the measurement of self-esteem is very relevant to social work research and practice.

In the social work literature, there is substantial evidence that high self-esteem is associated with positive outcomes. For homeless people, lower self-esteem relates to high depressive symptoms and poor health status (Diblasio & Belcher, 1993). Robinson (2000) found that among ethnic minority (i.e., African Caribbean) adolescents, higher self-esteem was related to positive racial identity attitudes. In a study examining the relationships between self-esteem instability and sexual be- havior among gay and bisexual men, Martin and Knox (1997) found that those who presented unstable self-esteem were more likely to report avoidance coping behaviors, loneliness, and lower social support compared to those whose self-esteem was relatively stable. In addition, individuals with unstable and lower self-esteem reportedly engaged more in risky sexual behaviors (e.g., unprotected sex with strangers).

Self-esteem has been found to be associated with welfare use. Kunz and Kalil (1999) found that individuals with lower self-esteem early in life were more likely to receive welfare (i.e., AFDC or TANF) by the age of 28, based on data from the National Longitudinal Survey of Youth. Savaya (1998) examined the associations between self-esteem and use of professional services among Arab women living in Israel and found that, on average, those who used professional services (e.g., doctor and hospital, prenatal care, mental health, family and marital counseling, employment, or social welfare) presented lower self-esteem than those who did not use these services. The self-esteem of those who received services from employment or social welfare agencies was especially low.

These findings from the social work literature suggest that self-esteem may be of critical interest for social workers because it is associated with individuals' psychological outcomes (e.g., depression, loneliness), social outcomes (e.g., social support), and behavior (e.g., sexual behavior or human services use). Social work research has focused on self-esteem as a key variable in evaluating the effectiveness of interventions. For example, in an evaluation of the long-term effectiveness of group counseling for women who were survivors of child sexual abuse, self-esteem was a major outcome variable (e.g., Bagley & Young, 1998).

The previously described social work literature on self-esteem utilized the Rosenberg Self-Esteem Scale (Rosenberg, 1965). Reflecting its position as a major measurement tool, the scale has been translated into American sign-language and its internal consistency has been assessed for individuals with hearing disabilities (Crowe, 2002). Consistent with its original development, the scale has been used by social work researchers as a unidimensional measure. However, recent research indicates that measures of global self-esteem combine two different dimensions–positive (i.e., self-enhancement) and negative (i.e., self-deprecation) (Owens, 1993, 1994). Owens (1993) argued that a more precise understanding of negative self-esteem in terms of its development and maintenance has been hindered because researchers tend to overemphasize global self-esteem. He offered empirical evidence of the two dimensions, showing the differential impact of negative and positive self-evaluations on emotional and social well-being among adolescents. For example, self-deprecation was strongly related to depression, whereas self-enhancement was not (Owens, 1994). By contrast, both self-deprecation and self-enhancement were related to adolescents' grades in school. Thus, correlates of the two dimensions of self-evaluation are not always the same. Despite its validated differential impact, sub-dimensions of global self-esteem have not been examined for social work clients and the validity of the two dimension self-esteem measure has not been tested among individuals with severe mental illness.

CURRENT STUDY

This study aims to address the gaps in previous social work literature–that is, the lack of studies testing the validity of the two-dimensional theory of self-esteem among social work clients. Participants in this study are individuals with serious mental illness, being served in psychosocial rehabilitation agencies. Due to deinstitutionalization, increasing numbers of individuals with mental illness seek services from community agencies, where social workers serve as the principal professional group providing mental health services (Stromwall, 2002). Individuals with mental illness experience various stresses related to their mental illness–not only symptoms but also the stigma of mental illness (Link et al., 1989, 1997) which often negatively influences their self-esteem (Link et al., 2001). Thus, in this study, we also consider the relationship of self-esteem to psychological, social, and behavioral variables for these individuals.

As a means of testing the validity of the two-dimensional self-esteem measure, this study first examines the factor structure of the 10-item Rosenberg Self-Esteem Scale (Rosenberg, 1965), through confirmatory factor analysis, to test the theory of bi-dimensional self-esteem (Owens, 1993, 1994). After analyzing the factor structure, we present bivariate associations of both the global self-esteem measure and the two dimensions of self-esteem with measures of socio-demographics, mental health, and behavioral coping styles to examine whether these self-esteem measures are differentially associated with relevant variables. Socio-demographic characteristics related to self-esteem in previous research, such as age (e.g., Robins et al., 2002), race (e.g., Gray-Little & Hafdahl, 2000), gender (e.g., Kling et al., 1999), and socio-economic status (e.g., income and education; Pinquart & Sorensen, 2000), are included. Mental health variables included are diagnosis and symptoms (Shern et al., 1994), service use (Kunz & Kalil, 1999), and causal attributions of mental illness (Alvidrez, 1999); the behavioral variables included are measures of coping styles–withdrawal and secrecy (Link et al., 1997).

The study then examines whether the factors predictive of global self-esteem differ from those predictive of the two dimensions of self-esteem, using multiple regression analyses. Analyses also examine whether factors predictive of the self-enhancement dimension differ from those predictive of the self-deprecation dimension. Finally, the effects of the two dimensions of self-esteem on behavioral coping styles are tested to examine whether the two dimensions differ from each other in predicting behavioral coping style.

METHODS

Sample and Data Collection

The sample consists of 461 individuals with serious mental illness (MI), recruited from 25 community-based psychosocial rehabilitation agencies (e.g., supported education programs, consumer drop-in centers, and clubhouse programs) in southeast Michigan, located within 70 miles of Ann Arbor. The data were collected through a survey administered in a small group-format at each agency. Each group was composed of 5 to 10 consumers. After informed consent was obtained, participants were given a training session about how to fill out the questionnaire. Participants completed practice questions using Likert scales, true/false, and open-ended questions. Immediately following the practice session, they began answering the actual survey. When they had questions, they were asked to raise their hands so that the researchers could respond. A total of 54 consumers were helped to some degree. Post hoc analyses indicated that, in terms of gender and race, those who received assistance did not differ from those who completed surveys for themselves. Participants' mean age was 44.47 (*SD* = 10.55) and 268 of the participants were male (58%). Three hundred participants were Caucasian (65%), 121 African American (26%), 19 American Indian/Alaskan native (4%), and nine were Asian/Pacific Islanders (2%). Approximately 28% of the participants (*n* = 133) reported an education level of less than high school, 29% (*n* = 134) high school or GED, and 43% (*n* = 194) reported more than high school. The self-reported mean duration of their mental illness was 21 years (*SD* = 11.90), and the average number of lifetime hospitalizations was about eight, with a median of four (*SD* = 12.12).

Measures

Measures were selected that showed acceptable reliability in previous research with individuals with MI. Cronbach alpha values, presented below, are for the current study sample and indicate that all measures hold acceptable levels of internal consistency. The mean scores reported are the mean item scores of a scale across the sample of respondents.

Socio-Demographic Variables

Age was calculated in years based on the birth date and the time of data collection ($M = 44.47$, $SD = 10.55$). *Race* was assessed following census definitions. For the analyses reported here, African Americans ($n = 121$, coded '1') were compared to all other races ($n = 340$). *Gender* was assessed as male ($n = 268$, coded '1') versus female ($n = 192$). *Education* was measured as the highest grade completed. For the analyses, participants with high school or GED and more than high school ($n = 328$, coded '1') were compared to those with an education level of less than high school ($n = 133$). *Monthly household income* included participants' earnings, the earnings of any others who lived with them, child support payments, and entitlements such as food stamps or SSI ($M = $1,665.25$, $SD = 5,090.12$, $Mdn = 647.00$). In order to deal with positive skew, log transformed values for this variable were used in the analyses.

Characteristics Related to Mental Health

Diagnosis was assessed by consumer self-report. A total of 160 (34.7%) consumers reported schizophrenia as their primary diagnosis, 52 (11.3%) schizoaffective disorder, 89 (19.3%) major depression, 81 (17.6%) bipolar disorder, 5 (1.1%) obsessive compulsive disorder, and 49 (10.6%) reported other diagnoses. Twenty-five (2%) consumers did not provide any specific diagnosis. For the analyses, depression (coded '1') was compared to all other diagnoses as the literature indicates that depressive symptoms are closely associated with self-esteem among individuals with severe mental illness (Shahar & Davidson, 2003).

Psychiatric symptoms were assessed using the 14-item Colorado Symptom Index (Shern, Wilson, Coen, Patrick, Foster, & Bartsch, 1994), which measures how often a person experiences emotional and psychiatric symptoms, such as anxiety, depression, and psychotic symptoms. Response options to the questions ranged from never (coded '1') to at least every day (coded '5') (M = 2.50, SD = 0.87, α = .87).

Service satisfaction was assessed using the 8-item Client Service Satisfaction Questionnaire (Cleary, 1981), which measures the extent to which individuals are satisfied with the mental health services they receive. Response options ranged from not at all ('1') to quite a bit ('4') (M = 2.93, SD = 0.60, α = .76).

Counts of service use were measured using 10 items from the Client Resource Use Questionnaire (Calsyn, 1993), which asks what types of services (e.g., psychiatric emergency service, inpatient psychiatric service, services in clubhouse or day treatment program, adult foster care, etc.) were received during the last three months. Responses were coded either yes ('1'), if a client used a service, or no ('0') if not. The count of yes answers (from 0 to 10) was used for the analysis (M = 3.20, SD = 1.97).

Individuals' beliefs about causes of mental illness were assessed using 16 items from the Opinions of Mental Illness Scale (Alvidrez, 1999), which measures how much individuals agree or disagree with statements about the causes of mental illness. Response options range from strongly disagree ('1') to strongly agree ('5'). Factor analyses produced two distinctive factors–i.e., *Cause of MI as Stressful Life Events* (M = 3.20, SD = 0.93, α = .86) (i.e., MI is caused by sexual abuse, physical abuse, traumatic events, physical illness, the deaths of loved ones, or having a difficult childhood) and *Cause of MI as Supernatural* (M = 2.36, SD = 0.90, α = .62) (i.e., MI is caused by God's will, bad luck or fate, weather, or having a weak character). Other factors were not included in the analysis because they had poor internal consistency.

Self-Esteem was assessed using the Rosenberg Self-Esteem scale (Rosenberg, 1965). Based on Owens (1993), the two subscales were: *Self-Enhancement* (M = 3.73, SD = 0.79, α = .82), including 5 items: (1) I feel that I am a person of worth, at least on an equal basis with others; (2) I feel that I have a number of good qualities; (3) I am able to do things as well as most people; (4) I take a positive attitude toward myself; (5) On the whole, I am satisfied with myself. *Self-Deprecation* (M = 2.79, SD = 0.89, α = .78) included these 5 items: (1) All in all, I am inclined to feel that I am a failure; (2) I feel that I do not have much to be proud of; (3) I wish I could have more respect for myself; (4) I certainly feel useless at times; and (5) At times, I think I am no good at all. Responses to questions ranged from strongly disagree ('1') to strongly agree ('5').

Behavioral coping styles were measured using two measures developed by Link and colleagues, with response options from strongly disagree ('1') to strongly agree ('5'). The *Behavioral Withdrawal Scale* (Link et al., 1989, 1997) contains 6 items measuring tendencies to withdraw from applying for a job, attending a school, and meeting friends to avoid mental illness disclosure ($M = 3.03$, $SD = .82$, $\alpha = 0.82$). The other measure of behavioral coping style, *Keeping MI Secret* (Link et al., 1989, 1997), contains 4 items that reflect the individual's tendency to keep his/her mental illness secret from others ($M = 3.24$, $SD = 0.84$, $\alpha = 0.75$).

Analyses

Confirmatory factor analyses used AMOS 4 (Arbuckle & Wothke. 1999). Specifically, two confirmatory factor analyses were carried out: one for a one-factor solution (i.e., the traditional usage of the Rosenberg Self-Esteem Scale) and the other for a two-factor solution (i.e., testing the two dimensions of self-esteem). Figures 1 and 2 present the hypothesized one- and two-factor models, respectively. Followed by the confirmatory factor analyses, tests on the changes in Chi-Square between the one-factor model and the two-factor model were performed to determine which model fits the data better. Bivariate analyses utilized Pearson Product Moment correlations, and multivariate analyses employed ordinary least squares multiple regression. The same variables were included in the bivariate and multivariate analyses. Bivariate analyses show simple zero-order correlations between two variables of interest. Multivariate regression analyses show the associations between two variables of interest (i.e., an independent variable and a dependent variable), controlling for the influences of other variables in the equation. Thus, multivariate analyses provide a control for Type I error which is more conservative than statistical adjustments such as Bonferroni correction.

RESULTS

Confirmatory Factor Analyses

Table 1 summarizes the results of confirmatory factor analyses, including standardized betas of factor coefficients and fit indices. It fur-

FIGURE 1. Hypothesized One-Factor Model

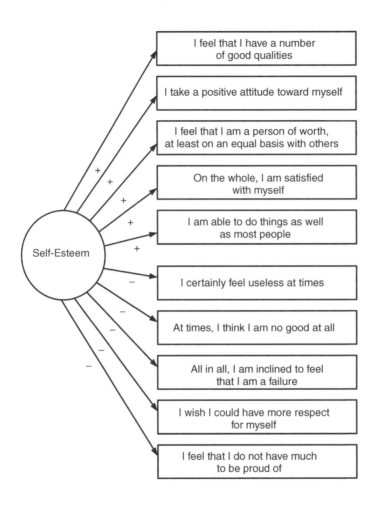

ther shows the results of a Chi-Square test between the one- and two-factor models. The model fit indices show that the two-factor solution (IFI = 0.99; RMSEA = 0.086; SRMR = 0.056) fits the data much better than the one-factor solution (IFI = 0.96; RMSEA = 0.174; SRMR = 0.113). Tests on the changes in Likelihood Ratio Chi-Square between the one-factor model ($\chi^2_{(35, n = 461)}$ = 521.43) and the two-factor model ($\chi^2_{(34, n = 461)}$ = 150.77) also indicate that the two-factor model fits the

FIGURE 2. Hypothesized Two-Factor Model

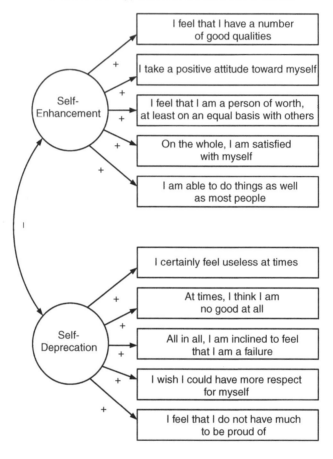

data significantly better than the one-factor model ($LR\chi^2_{(1, n = 461)} = 370.66, p < 0.000$).

Results of Bivariate Correlations

Bivariate correlational analyses examined the relationships between self-esteem and variables of interest (i.e., socio-demographics, mental health, and behavioral coping); results are summarized in Table 2. With regard to the relationship between the global self-esteem measure and variables of interest, age ($r = .10$), household income ($r = .14$), and ser-

TABLE 1. The Results of Confirmatory Factor Analyses: Comparisons Between One-Factor Solution and Two-Factor Solution

Self-esteem items	One-factor Solution Standardized B	Two-factor Solution Standardized B	
	Self-esteem	SW[a]	SD[b]
I feel that I have a number of good qualities	.56	.68	
I take a positive attitude toward myself	.66	.75	
I feel that I am a person of worth, at least on an equal basis with others	.62	.69	
On the whole, I am satisfied with myself	.70	.72	
I am able to do things as well as most people	.61	.65	
I certainly feel useless at times	−.59		.80
At times, I think I am no good at all	−.61		.84
All in all, I am inclined to feel that I am a failure	−.64		.69
I wish I could have more respect for myself	−.30		.42
I feel that I do not have much to be proud of	−.42		.45
Covariance between SW and SD	N/A	−.31	
Model Fits			
Chi-square	$\chi^2_{(35, n=461)} = 521.43$	$\chi^2_{(34, n=461)} = 150.77$	
IFI[c]	.96	.99	
RMSEA[d]	1.74 (.161 < CI < .187)	8.06 (.073 < CI < .101)	
SRMR[e] (n = 393)	0.113	0.056	

Notes: a. Self-Worth
b. Self-Deprecation
c. Incremental Fit Index
d. Root-Mean Square Error of Approximation
e. Standardized Root-Mean Residual

vice satisfaction ($r = .13$) were positively correlated with global self-esteem. In addition, depression diagnosis ($r = −.11$), psychiatric symptoms ($r = −.51$), belief in causes of MI as stressful life events ($r = −.12$), and beliefs in causes of MI as supernatural ($r = −.15$) were negatively correlated with the one-dimensional self-esteem. Both behavioral coping measures were negatively correlated with self-esteem, indicating that individuals with higher self-esteem had lower levels of behavioral withdrawal ($r = −.17$), and were less likely to keep MI secret ($r = −.30$).

TABLE 2. Results of Bivariate Correlations

	One-Dimension	Two-Dimensions	
	Total Self-esteem	Self-enhancement	Self-deprecation
Socio-demographic characteristics			
1	.10*	.08	−.10*
2	.05	.06	−.03
3	.01	.05	.03
4	.08	.03	−.10*
5	.14**	.12*	−.12*
Mental health background			
6	−.11*	−.06	.12*
7	−.51**	−.37**	.49**
8	.13**	.17**	−.05
9	−.09	−.04	.10*
10	−.12**	−.01	.19**
11	−.15**	−.02	.22**
Behavioral Copings			
12	−.17**	−.25**	.05
13	−.30**	−.18**	.32**

$*p \leq .05; **p \leq .01$

Notes:
  1. Age
  2. Race (1 = Black)
  3. Gender (1 = Male)
  4. Education (1 = high school and higher)
  5. Household income (Log-transformation was done to fix distribution problem)
  6. Diagnosis (1 = Depression)
  7. Psychiatric symptoms
  8. Service satisfaction
  9. Counts of service use
  10. Causes of MI as stressful life events
  11. Causes of MI as supernatural causes
  12. Behavioral withdrawals
  13. Keeping MI secret

The results of the correlation analyses for self-enhancement were not the same as the results for self-deprecation. Self-enhancement was positively correlated with household income ($r = .12$) and with service satisfaction ($r = .17$), and negatively correlated with psychiatric symptoms ($r = -.37$), behavioral withdrawal ($r = -.25$), and keeping MI secret ($r = -.18$). Self-deprecation was correlated with more variables than was self-enhancement. Age ($r = -.10$), education ($r = -.10$), and household income ($r = -.12$) were negatively correlated with self-deprecation. Self-deprecation was positively correlated with depression diagnosis ($r =$

.12), psychiatric symptoms ($r = .49$), counts of service use ($r = .10$), be-liefs about causes of MI as stressful life events ($r = .19$), beliefs about causes of MI as supernatural ($r = .22$), and keeping MI secret ($r = .32$).

Results of Multivariate Regression Analyses

Regression analyses first examined whether the socio-demographic and mental health predictors of the three self-esteem measures (i.e., global self-esteem, self-enhancement, and self-deprecation) differed; the results are summarized in Table 3. Standardized betas are reported. The regression analysis explained about 29% of the variance in global self-esteem ($R^2 = .29$). Specifically, age ($\beta = .13$) and income ($\beta = .14$) were positively associated with global self-esteem, indicating older in-dividuals and individuals with higher education have higher global self-esteem. However, race, gender, and education were not signifi-cantly associated with global self-esteem. Controlling for socio-demo-graphic characteristics, individuals with depression diagnosis ($\beta = -.12$), more psychiatric symptoms ($\beta = -.52$), and lower satisfaction with services ($\beta = .13$) had lower self-esteem.

Variables in the regression explained about 17% of variance in self-enhancement ($R^2 = .17$). Older individuals ($\beta = .11$) and those with more income ($\beta = .13$) reported higher self-enhancement. Controlling for socio-demographic characteristics, individuals with more psychiat-ric symptoms ($\beta = -.37$) and those less satisfied with services ($\beta = .15$) presented lower levels of self-enhancement. Controlling for socio-de-mographic variables, individuals who believed in causes of MI as stressful life events presented marginally higher self-enhancement ($\beta = .09$); belief about causes of MI as supernatural was not significantly as-sociated with self-enhancement.

As shown in Table 3, the variables of interest explained about 30% of the variance in self-deprecation ($R^2 = .30$). Specifically, older individu-als ($\beta = -.11$) and individuals with more income ($\beta = -.11$) showed lower levels of self-deprecation. Controlling for socio-demographic variables, higher levels of self-deprecation were significantly associated with depres-sion diagnosis ($\beta = .13$), more psychiatric symptoms ($\beta = .50$), and belief in causes of MI as supernatural ($\beta = .10$).

The second set of regression analyses examined whether self-en-hancement differed from self-deprecation in predicting the two behav-ioral coping variables. Table 4 summarizes the results. Controlling for

TABLE 3. Results of Regression Analyses: Factors Associated with Self-Esteem

	One-Dimension	Two-Dimensions	
	Total Self-esteem	Self-enhancement	Self-deprecation
	Standardized B	Standardized B	Standardized B
Socio-demographic characteristics			
1	.13*	.11*	−.11*
2	.03	.06	−.00
3	−.02	.08	.03
4	.05	.02	−.07
5	.14**	.13*	−.11*
Mental health background			
6	−.12**	−.06	.13**
7	−.51***	−.37***	.50***
8	.12**	.15**	−.05
9	.01	.02	.03
10	.04	.09^	.02
11	−.02	.07	.10*
12. R^2	.29	.17	.30

^$p ≤ .10$; *$p ≤ .05$; **$p ≤ .01$; ***$p ≤ .001$

Notes:
1. Age
2. Race (1 = Black)
3. Gender (1 = Male)
4. Education (1 = high school and higher)
5. Household income (Log-transformation was done to fix distribution problem)
6. Diagnosis (1 = Depression)
7. Psychiatric symptoms
8. Service satisfaction
9. Counts of service use
10. Causes of MI as stressful life events
11. Causes of MI as stressful supernatural causes
12. Adjusted R^2

socio-demographic and mental health variables, self-enhancement was negatively associated with behavioral withdrawal ($β = −.26$), indicating that individuals with higher self-enhancement were less likely to withdraw. Self-enhancement was not significantly associated with keeping MI secret. By contrast, self-deprecation was positively associated with keeping MI secret ($β = .21$), but not significantly associated with behavioral withdrawal.

TABLE 4. Results of Regression Analyses: Self-Esteem Predicting Behavioral Coping

	Behavioral Copings	
	Behavioral Withdrawals	Keeping MI Secret
	Standardized B	Standardized B
Socio-demographic characteristics		
1	.02	−.09^
2	−.04	.04
3	−.04	−.03
4	.00	.02
5	−.11*	.02
Mental health background		
6	.02	.07
7	.06	.27***
8	−.05	.02
9	.08	−.01
10	−.15*	.13*
11	−.03	−.03
Two dimensions of self-esteem		
12	−.26***	−.07
13	−.01	.21**
14. R^2	.07	.13

^$p \le .10$; *$p \le .05$; **$p \le .01$; ***$p \le .001$

Notes:
1. Age
2. Race (1 = Black)
3. Gender (1 = Male)
4. Education (1 = high school and higher)
5. Household income (Log-transformation was done to fix distribution problem)
6. Diagnosis (1 = Depression)
7. Psychiatric symptoms
8. Service satisfaction
9. Counts of service use
10. Causes of MI as stressful life events
11. Causes of MI as supernatural causes
12. Self-enhancement
13. Self-deprecation
14. Adjusted R^2

DISCUSSION

The purpose of the study was to test the validity of the two-dimensional self-esteem model (Owens, 1993) for individuals with mental illness, by examining whether the factor structure of Rosenberg's (1965) Self-Esteem Scale consists of two dimensions and whether the two dimensions of self-esteem are associated with different predictive factors and behavioral outcomes. The results of factor analyses indicated that the traditional self-esteem scale does reflect two dimensions–self-enhancement and self-deprecation. In order to examine how the two dimensions of self-esteem are differently associated with variables of interest, bivariate correlations and multivariate regression analyses were conducted. Results of the correlational and regression analyses showed that factors significantly associated with self-enhancement differ from factors associated with self-deprecation. The findings of factor analyses, bivariate analyses, and multivariate analyses all support the two dimensions of self-esteem theory (Owens, 1993, 1994), indicating that social work researchers and practitioners should be more selective in using the traditional Rosenberg Self-Esteem Scale.

Bivariate Correlates of Self-Esteem Measures

Supporting the two dimensions of self-esteem theory, the bivariate correlations of the three self-esteem measures differ from each other. Among the socio-demographic variables, different correlations were found for age. Older individuals presented higher global self-esteem than younger individuals, consistent with previous findings among adults aged 20 to 60 (Robins et al., 2002). Although older individuals did not differ from younger in self-enhancement, they showed significantly lower self-deprecation, suggesting that negative self-evaluations among individuals may decrease with age (or there could be a cohort effect). Previous findings of significant age differences in global self-esteem might have been primarily caused by the age difference in self-deprecation.

In mental health background variables (diagnosis, service satisfaction, counts of service use, and beliefs in causes of MI), different correlation results were also found. Individuals with higher global self-esteem were more likely to have non-depression diagnosis, to have fewer psychiatric symptoms, to be more satisfied with services. They were also less likely to endorse beliefs that MI is caused by stressful life events as well as beliefs of its causes in the supernatural. It is interesting to note that self-enhancement was related to fewer mental health variables than self-esteem–being associated only with psychiatric symptoms and with service satisfaction. By contrast, self-deprecation was associated with more mental health variables than self-enhancement. Specifically, individuals with higher self-deprecation were more likely to have depression diagnoses, to have more psychiatric symptoms, to use a greater number of services, and to endorse beliefs that MI is caused by stressful life events as well as beliefs that its causes are in the supernatural.

The findings suggest that individuals who frequently use mental health services are likely to evaluate themselves negatively, which is consistent with previous findings (e.g., Savaya, 1998). Both measures reflecting beliefs in causes of MI were negatively associated with global self-esteem. Although self-enhancement did not significantly vary by beliefs in causes of MI, individuals who more strongly believed causes of MI to be either stressful life events or supernatural presented significantly higher self-deprecation. This finding indicates that cognitive understanding of causes of mental illness is more strongly associated with self-deprecation than with self-enhancement.

In the coping domain, different correlation patterns were found for the behavioral withdrawal variable. Individuals with higher self-enhancement were less likely to present behavioral withdrawal, whereas self-deprecation was not significantly correlated with behavioral withdrawal. This finding, that individuals with higher self-esteem or self-enhancement are less likely to behaviorally withdraw, is consistent with the findings of previous stigma literature (Link et al., 1989, 1997).

Multivariate Correlates of Self-Esteem Measures

Controlling for socio-demographic characteristics, differential multivariate relationships with the self-esteem measures were found for diagnosis, service satisfaction, and both of the variables reflecting beliefs in causes of MI. The associations with diagnosis and service satisfaction are consistent with the findings of the bivariate analyses. That is, individuals with depression diagnosis presented greater self-deprecation than those with other diagnoses. Further, individuals with greater service satisfaction presented higher self-esteem and higher self-enhancement.

It is interesting to note that "causes of MI as stressful life events" was associated only with self-enhancement–those who believed that stressful life events are the primary causes of mental illness presented marginally higher self-enhancement scores. Given that stressful life events are often controllable, higher self-enhancement being associated with such beliefs is understandable. By contrast, those who believe in supernatural causes of mental illness are more likely to have high self-deprecation. Given that supernatural causes (e.g., God's will, fate, etc.) are hard to control, such a belief might lead to higher self-deprecation or, in contrast, feelings of self-deprecation might produce rationalizations of mental illness being uncontrollable.

Further analyses examined the relationships between the two dimensions of self-esteem and behavioral coping after controlling for socio-demographics and mental health background variables. Again, supporting the two-dimensional theory of self-esteem (Owens, 1993), self-enhancement was found to differ from self-deprecation in predicting behavioral coping. Specifically, individuals with higher self-enhancement were less likely to engage in behavioral withdrawal; however, keeping MI secret did not vary by self-enhancement. By contrast, individuals with greater self-deprecation were more likely to keep their history of MI secret, but behavioral withdrawal did not vary by self-deprecation.

Validity of the Self-Esteem Measures

Bivariate and multivariate analyses provide some evidence as to the validity of the two self-esteem measures. Some significant correlates (i.e., household income, psychiatric symptoms, and keeping MI secret) of the global self-esteem scale were also found to be significantly correlated with both self-enhancement and self-deprecation (indicating the convergent validity of the two dimensions of self-esteem). However, other correlates of the global self-esteem scale were not correlated with self-enhancement but with self-deprecation (i.e., age, diagnosis, and both measures of beliefs in causes of MI), while others failed to correlate with self-deprecation but did correlate with self-enhancement (i.e., service satisfaction and behavioral withdrawals). Furthermore, there were some variables which did not correlate with the global self-esteem scale but did correlate with self-deprecation (i.e., education and counts of service use). These differing correlates support the divergent validity of the two dimensions of self-esteem, which suggests that the two measures of self-esteem are different from the global self-esteem measure and worthy of separate analysis.

The results of multivariate analyses also support the convergent and divergent validity of the two self-esteem measures with global self-esteem. That is, several variables (i.e., age, household income, and psychiatric symptoms) were predictive of the global self-esteem as well as of self-enhancement and self-deprecation, supporting the convergent validity of the two dimensions of self-esteem scales as tools for measuring the self. By contrast, causes of MI variables were not associated with global self-esteem, but with either self-enhancement or self-deprecation, supporting divergent validity. With regard to the predictors of self-esteem and self-deprecation, age, household income, and psychiatric symptoms were associated with both constructs, indicating convergent validity. By contrast, service satisfaction and causes of MI as stressful life events were associated only with self-enhancement, whereas diagnosis and causes of MI as supernatural were associated only with self-deprecation. Further, self-enhancement was predictive of behavioral withdrawals, whereas self-deprecation was predictive of secrecy behavior. These findings of differing associations also indicate the divergent validity of self-enhancement and self-deprecation, suggesting self-enhancement and self-deprecation are importantly different constructs.

Implications for Social Work

Deinstitutionalization has increased the number of consumers living in communities as well as community-based psychosocial rehabilitation service agencies (Segal, 1995). These services aim to promote more effective adaptation to society for individuals with psychiatric disabilities (Silverstein, 2000) by providing rehabilitation services to enhance consumers' social and vocational skills, assuming that achieving higher education (Mowbray, Collins, & Bybee, 1999) and/or obtaining appropriate employment (Mueser, Becker, Torrey et al., 1997) or meaningful daytime activities are essential for successful rehabilitation. Appropriate behavioral styles are also critical to successful rehabilitation. For example, an extremely withdrawn person often lacks motivation to attend school or to get a job; and a person who keeps his/her mental illness history rigidly secret is not likely to get proper rehabilitation services. Link and colleagues (2001) suggest that self-esteem interventions could be effective in reducing the negative effects of stigma associated with MI by modifying inappropriate behavioral styles.

This study showed that different behavioral styles are associated with different dimensions of self-esteem. When social workers intervene to modify behavioral styles, our findings suggest the need to select target areas of self-esteem, depending on specific behaviors. For example, social workers can select self-deprecation as a target area when a consumer overly engages in keeping MI secret. By contrast, when a consumer presents inappropriate behavioral withdrawal, social workers may select self-enhancement as a target for intervention. After deciding on the target area (e.g., self-enhancement or self-deprecation), specific interventions could productively be based on associated factors such as, for increased self-enhancement, reduced psychiatric symptoms, increased service satisfaction, or education about the causes of MI. By contrast, social workers might try to reduce depressive symptoms or to educate consumers about the causes of MI when self-deprecation is the target.

CONCLUSION

The limitations of this study should be acknowledged. This study relied on a convenience sample of community-living individuals with mental illness derived from psychosocial rehabilitation service agencies in a certain geographic area. This specific sample limits the scope of generalizability of the findings to other populations, such as psychiatric inpatients or possibly individuals with MI in different areas. Another limitation is that this study utilized a cross-sectional design. Certain domains of behavioral outcomes may influence psychological characteristics and self-esteem; however, a cross-sectional design cannot examine these possible multi-directional relationships. This study used self-reported diagnoses, which undermines the validity of the diagnosis measure. Finally, it should also be acknowledged that the data collection method employed for the study (e.g., self-administration, allowing consumers to ask questions when they have problems answering) could introduce bias into individuals' responses. Future studies should address these limitations.

Regardless of the limitations, the findings of the current study are notable. The significance of the study lies in its examination of the factor structure of the Rosenberg Self-Esteem Scale which has been used as a unidimensional measure in most previous research. A contribution of the current study is to broaden the understanding of self-esteem by validating the two-dimensional theory of self-esteem (Owens, 1993, 1994) among individuals with mental illness, served by psychosocial rehabilitation agencies. By identifying the dimensions that underlie the traditional self-esteem scale, this study suggests that it may be more useful for social work practitioners and researchers to employ a two-dimensional rather than a global approach to studying and understanding self-esteem (Owens, 1994).

REFERENCES

Alvidrez, J. (1999). Ethnic variations in mental health attitudes and service use among low-income African American, Latina, and European American young women. *Community Mental Health Journal, 35*(6), 515-530.

Arbuckle, J. L., & Wothke, W. (1999). *Amos 4.0 User's Guide.* Chicago, IL: Small Waters Corporation.

Bagley, C., & Young, L. (1998). Long-term evaluation of group counseling for women with a history of child sexual abuse: Focus on depression, self-esteem, suicidal behaviors, and social support. *Social Work with Groups, 21*(3), 63-74.

Calsyn, R. J. (1993). Prediction perceived service need, service awareness, and service utilization. *Journal of Gerontological Social Work, 21*, 59-76.

Carver, C. S., Scheier, M., & Weinstraub, J. K. (1989). Assessing coping strategies: A theoretically based approach. *Journal of Personality & Social Psychology, 56*, 267-283.

Cleary, P. J. (1981). Problems of internal consistency and scaling in life event schedules. *Journal of Psychosomatic Research, 25*(4), 309-320.

Crocker, J., & Wolfe, C. T. (2001). Contingencies of self-worth. *Psychological Review: Special Issue, 108*, 593-623.

Crowe, T. V. (2002). Translation of the Rosenberg Self-Esteem Scale into American sign language: A principal components analysis. *Social Work Research, 26*(1), 57-63.

Diblasio, F. A., & Belcher, J. R. (1993). Social work outreach to homeless people and the need to address issues of self-esteem. *Health & Social Work, 18*(4), 281-287.

Gray-Little, B., & Hafdahl, A. R. (2000). Factors influencing racial comparisons of self-esteem: A quantitative review. *Psychological Bulletin, 126*, 26-54.

Kling, K. C., Hyde, J. S., Sowers, C. J., & Buswell, B. N. (1999). Gender differences in self-esteem: A meta-analysis. *Psychological Bulletin, 125*, 470-500.

Kunz, J., & Kalil, A. (1999). Self-esteem, self-efficacy, and welfare use. *Social Work Research, 23*(2), 119-126.

Lazarus, R. S., & Folkman, S. (1984). *Stress, appraisal, and coping.* New York: Springer.

Link, B. G., Cullen, F. T., Struening, E., Shrout, P. E., & Dohrenwend, B. P. (1989). A modified labeling theory approach to mental disorders: An empirical assessment. *American Sociological Review, 54*, 400-423.

Link, B. G., Struening, E. L., Neese-Todd, A. S., & Phelan, J. C. (2001). The consequences of stigma for the self-esteem of people with mental illnesses. *Psychiatric Services, 52*, 1621-1625.

Link, B. G., Struenig, E. L., Rahav, M., Phelan, J. C., & Nuttbrock, L. (1997). On stigma and its consequences: Evidence from a longitudinal study of men with dual diagnoses of mental illness and substance abuse. *Journal of Health & Social Behavior, 38*, 177-190.

Martin, J. I., & Knox, J. (1997). Self-esteem instability and its implications for HIV prevention among gay men. *Health & Social Work, 22*(4), 264-273.

Mowbray, C. T., Collins, M. E., & Bybee, D. (1999). Supported education for individuals with psychiatric disabilities: Long-term outcome from an experimental study. *Social Work Research, 23*(2), 89-100.

Mueser, K. T., Becker, D. R., Torrey, W. C., Xie, H., Bond, G. R., Drake, R. E., & Dain, B. J. (1997). Work and nonvocational domains of functioning in persons with severe mental illness: A longitudinal analysis. *Journal of Nervous & Mental Disease*, *185*(7), 419-426.

Owens, T. J. (1993). Accentuate the positive and the negative: Rethinking the use of self-esteem, self-deprecation, and self-confidence. *Social Psychology Quarterly*, *56*, 288-299.

Owens, T. J. (1994). Two dimensions of self-esteem: Reciprocal effects of positive self-worth and self-deprecation on adolescent problems. *American Sociological Review*, *59*, 391-407.

Pearlin, L. L. (1989). The sociological study of stress. *Journal of Health & Social Behavior*, *30*, 241-256.

Petty, R. E., Wegener, D. T., & Fabrigar, L. F. (1997). Attitudes and attitude change. *Annual Review of Psychology*, *48*, 609-647.

Pinquart, M., & Sorensen, S. (2000). Influences of socioeconomic status, social network, and competence on subjective well-being in later life: A meta-analysis. *Psychology and Aging*, *15*(2), 187-224.

Robins, R. W., Trzesniewski, K. H., Tracy, J. L., Gosling, S. D., & Potter, J. (2002). Global self-esteem across the life span. *Psychology and Aging*, *17*(3), 423-434.

Robinson, L. (2000). Racial identity attitudes and self-esteem of black adolescents in residential care: An exploratory study. *British Journal of Social Work*, *30*(1), 3-24.

Rosenberg, M. (1965). *Society and the adolescent self-image*. Princeton, NJ: Princeton University Press.

Savaya, R. (1998). Associations among economic need, self-esteem, and Israeli Arab women's attitudes toward and use of professional services. *Social Work*, *43*(5), 445-454.

Segal, S. P. (1995). Deinstitutionalization. *Encyclopedia of Social Work, 19th Ed., Vol. 1*, 704-712.

Shahar, G., & Davidson, L. (2003). Depressive symptoms erode self-esteem in severe mental illness: A three-wave, cross-lagged study. *Journal of Consulting & Clinical Psychology*, *71*(5), 890-900.

Shern, D., Wilson, N., Coen, A., Patrick, D., Foster, M., & Bartsch, D. (1994). Client outcomes II: Longitudinal client data from the Colorado Treatment Outcome Study. *Milbank Quarterly*, *72*, 123-148.

Silverstein, S. M. (2000). Psychiatric rehabilitation of schizophrenia: Unsolved issues, current trends, and future direction. *Applied & Preventive Psychology*, *9*, 227-248.

Stromwall, L. K. (2002). Is social work's door open to people recovering from psychiatric disabilities? *Social Work*, *47*(1), 75-83.

Woolfolk, R. L., Novalany, J., Gara, M. A., Allen, L. A., & Polino, M. (1995). Self-complexity, self-evaluation, and depression: An examination of form and content within the self-schema. *Journal of Personality & Social Psychology*, *68*, 1108-1120.

The Child's View of Neighborhood:
Assessing a Neglected Element
in Direct Social Work Practice

Nicole Nicotera

SUMMARY. The research presented in this paper contributes to the social work profession by uncovering the child-neighborhood relationship as an element for assessment in direct social work practice. Neighborhood is often viewed as the domain of macro level practice. However, in direct social work practice, aspects of the broader social and physical environment are often omitted. The results of this qualitative study, in which 59 fourth and fifth graders were queried about their neighborhoods, indicate that the child-neighborhood relationship be viewed as a vital facet in direct practice assessments. Specifically, the findings suggest that four distinct components be included in the assessment of child-neighborhood relationships. Implications for the inclusion of

Nicole Nicotera, MSW, PhD, is Assistant Professor, Graduate School of Social Work, University of Denver, 2148 South High Street, Denver, CO 80208 (E-mail: nnicoter@du. edu).

Data for this study were drawn from a larger study that comprises dissertation research completed at the University of Washington, School of Social Work, Seattle, WA.

The author would like to acknowledge the support and guidance of her dissertation committee, Gunnar Almgren, PhD (Chair), Lewayne Gilchrist, PhD, and Susan P. Kemp, PhD.

[Haworth co-indexing entry note]: "The Child's View of Neighborhood: Assessing a Neglected Element in Direct Social Work Practice." Nicotera, Nicole. Co-published simultaneously in *Journal of Human Behavior in the Social Environment* (The Haworth Social Work Practice Press, an imprint of The Haworth Press, Inc.) Vol. 11, No. 3/4, 2005, pp. 105-133; and: *Approaches to Measuring Human Behavior in the Social Environment* (ed: William R. Nugent) The Haworth Social Work Practice Press, an imprint of The Haworth Press, Inc., 2005, pp. 105-133. Single or multiple copies of this article are available for a fee from The Haworth Document Delivery Service [1-800-HAWORTH, 9:00 a.m. - 5:00 p.m. (EST). E-mail address: docdelivery@haworthpress.com].

Available online at http://www.haworthpress.com/web/JHBSE
doi:10.1300/J137v11n03_06

neighborhood in bio-psycho-social assessments with children are discussed. *[Article copies available for a fee frm The Haworth Document Delivery Service: 1-800-HAWORTH. E-mail address: <docdelivery@haworthpress.com> Website: <http://www.HaworthPress.com> © 2005 by The Haworth Press, Inc. All rights reserved.]*

KEYWORDS. Neighborhood, physical environment, children, child-focused practice, social support, qualitative methods

This article explores assessment issues related to the application of the construct "neighborhood" in direct social work practice with children. The results of a qualitative research study in which neighborhood is measured and assessed through the lens of childhood are presented. The article begins with a discussion of the neglected, but significant construct "neighborhood" as it applies to social work practice. This discussion is followed by a review of literature, from several disciplines, that underscores the importance of neighborhoods in the lives of children. Next, the study methodology and results are presented. The concluding discussion examines the implications of the study results for assessing the construct "neighborhood" in social work practice with children.

The person-in-environment (PIE) framework, a hallmark of social work practice, compels social workers to provide assessments and interventions that are aimed at many levels of an individual's life from micro to macro. The Human Behavior in the Social Environment (HBSE) curriculum strives to provide students with opportunities to develop an understanding of human development in the context of the micro-macro continuum. However, in direct social work practice, aspects of the broader social and physical environment are often omitted. In fact, Kemp, Whittacker, and Tracy (1997, p. xi) note that a "long-neglected dimension in social work and human services practice is accurate environmental assessment and strategic environmental intervention." For various historical and contemporary reasons, social work assessments and interventions are frequently focused on individuals and their "choices," as if choices were made in a context-less vacuum. Behavioral assessments based on individualistic frameworks lack consideration of the role played by environmental context and the availability of resources within that context as dictated by a social-political structure founded on hierarchies of economics, skin color, language, gender, sexuality, and culture.

The dearth of attention on the assessment of neighborhoods in direct social work practice may result, in part, from the fact that traditional methods for neighborhood assessment, which are based on census data, do not readily lend themselves for use in direct social work practice. For example, census data provide strong indicators of the structural and demographic elements of a neighborhood, but these data alone do not account for the assessment of neighborhood social processes (Brooks-Gunn, Duncan, & Aber, 1997; Burton & Price-Spratlen, 1999; Tienda, 1991). However, the substance of assessment and intervention in direct social work practice resides within social processes. The scarcity of tools for the assessment of neighborhood social processes, related to the strengths and challenges in the lives of children, has resulted in the omission of neighborhood as a useful element in direct social work practice.

In addition to being sites of social processes, neighborhoods are also physical environments with which children must, for good or for ill, contend. Traditional census data assessments of neighborhood do not account for the physical conditions within them. However, various researchers (Moore, 1986; Lynch, 1979; Perkins, Meeks, & Taylor, 1992; Skejaeveland & Garling ,1997; Taylor, Wiley, Kuo, & Sullivan, 1998) report studies which confirm the influence of neighborhood physical environments on human behavior. These environments not only influence human actions and interactions, they also have some bearing on one's subjective experiences of self-in-place. Sutton (1996) elucidates this physical environment-subjectivity connection when she states, "places not only sustain individuals in a tangible way by providing shelter for various public and private activities, they tacitly communicate a way of life" (p. xiii). Halpern (1995) provides an example of this when he states, "ever since the 1950s the press, radio, and television have not hesitated to remind Cabrini Green (a Chicago public housing project) residents that the place they call home is a slum . . . the mass media has shaped the image of the Cabrini Green neighborhood as much as the residents themselves. By the 1960s the residents of the project neighborhoods were internalizing what the media said about them and were belittling themselves" (p. 79). Proshansky, Fabian, and Kaminoff (1983) echo the subjective nature of physical environments to which Halpern refers when they point out that the residents of a locale experience both the "physical reality" of that locality as well as the "social meanings and beliefs attached to it by those who live outside of it as well as its residents" (p. 62). In summary, assessment tools that can be utilized in direct social work practice need to incorporate the social processes and the physical conditions of neighborhoods as well as account for the subjective experiences of those who reside within them.

In addition, social work practitioners may overlook neighborhoods as a potential resource in the lives of children because a great deal of the literature on neighborhoods is framed in a deficit orientation (Brodsky, 1996; Coulton, Korbin, Su, & Chow, 1995; Crane, 1991; Sampson & Groves, 1989; Simcha-Fagin & Schwartz, 1986). Also, due to the scarcity of social work research on neighborhoods, one must investigate other disciplines such as environmental psychology, geography, sociology, and urban planning for knowledge about neighborhoods. Therefore, the practice application and strength-based lens of social work is absent from much of the literature on neighborhoods.

This absence, however, does not diminish the importance of environments in the lives of the children we serve and teach our students to serve. For example, Garbarino, Galambos, Plantz, and Kostenly (1992) discuss the significance of neighborhood environments for child development. They note, "The neighborhood in which the child lives is an early and major arena for exploration and social interaction, and serves as setting for the physical and emotional development of the child" (Garbarino et al., 1992, 202). In addition, David and Weinstein (1987) suggest that the following developmental outcomes are impacted by the physical environment:

1. Personal identity via the messages a person gets from visual cues in the environment as well as how people talk about those cues;
2. Competence via opportunities to develop mastery and control;
3. Cognitive, social, and motor skills via opportunities to explore a rich and varied environment;
4. Security and trust from access to predictable, comfortable surroundings with opportunities to socialize and have privacy.

Two other researchers underscore the process by which the outcomes noted above might result from child/physical environment transactions. Moore (1986) notes that play opportunities that enhance the development of competence are important for children. She suggests that neighborhood physical environments that present ubiquitous obstacles to play and exploration will limit a child's attainment of mastery and competence unless special care is taken to provide opportunities outside of the neighborhood. Additionally, Rivlin (1987) states that "every relationship is inextricably a component of a complex environmental system in which the human process and the setting define the meaning of the experience to the person" (p. 9). She notes the different messages about worthiness and ability to control the present and the future that are reflected to those who reside in the context of a middle-class home versus a homeless shelter, as well as the impact each setting would have on parenting and access to resources and services that promote parenting. She suggests that "each reality (the physical and social context in which a child resides) deposits its powerful experiences that become incorporated into children's conceptions of themselves and those around them" (Rivlin 1987, 10). Hence, neighborhoods have the potential to play an important role in the lives of children, yet the assessment of the child-neighborhood relationship is often omitted in direct social work practice. The significance of the neighborhood in the lives of children is examined further in the following literature review.

REVIEW OF LITERATURE

The literature that forms the foundation of our knowledge about neighborhoods and their influence in the lives of children arises from a variety of disciplines that include: architecture and urban planning, community psychology, environment psychology, geography, social work and sociology. Curiously, while children are the target population of much of the theory and research on neighborhoods, their views and experiences have often been peripheral in these endeavors. While there are a few exceptions (e.g., Bryant, 1985; Burton & Price-Spratlen, 1999; Hart, 1979; Moore, 1986; Nicotera, 2003; Sutton, 1992), a great many researchers have presumed knowledge of children's neighborhood experiences from the foundation of structural and demographic information about the neighborhoods where they reside. In light of this, the literature reviewed here focuses on studies that incorporate the lived neighborhood experiences of children. This focus is most relevant to social work practice with children as it uncovers the neighborhood experiences of children who may be similar to those we endeavor to assist. These studies also provide examples of various tools that could be utilized by social work practitioners for gathering information from children about their neighborhoods.

One of the more recent studies of child-neighborhood interactions (Lewis & Osofsky, 1997) reports on children's drawings about their neighborhoods in a moderate size, southern (USA) city. Children in the study were between the ages of 8 and 12 and all of them were African Americans who resided in low-income neighborhoods, some of which were known for high rates of violence. Children were asked to draw two pictures, one of their neighborhood and the second of what goes on in their neighborhood. In general, 9% percent of the children included depictions of violence in response to the general question "draw a picture of your neighborhood" while more than 60% of the children drew pictures that portrayed violence when drawing in response to the question, "what goes on in your neighborhood?" (Lewis & Osofsky, 1997).

The researchers defined violence in the drawings as "an act or behavior that causes damage or injury, or human figures engaged in verbal threats or activity labeled as fighting, hitting, or someone starting a fire or robbery" (Lewis & Osofsky 1997, 283). One eight-year-old boy drew a picture that portrays one girl shooting another girl, a rectangular shape labeled "drugs," and a person in a car. The child's caption on the picture read, "A girl shot a other girl" (Lewis & Osofsky, 1997, 284). Another child (age and gender not noted) drew a picture titled "Killing/Drugs" that depicts one person shooting another person. A third picture depicts a person labeled "Lady" who is saying, "Don't cry run" (Lewis & Osofsky, 1997, 287).

This study suggests that requests of children to draw "what goes on" in their neighborhoods, as opposed to the simpler query, "draw a picture of your neighborhood," will result in more detailed information about a neighborhood. This is useful information for child-focused social work practitioners. While the children's drawings presented in the Lewis and Osofsky (1997) study are enlightening, it is difficult to comprehend from drawings alone how neighborhood environments may influence the meanings that children make for themselves and the world around them. Therefore, while drawings by a child of her or his neighborhood are a useful tool for assessment in direct social work practice, they do not paint the full picture of the child-neighborhood relationship. I turn now to studies that provide more detailed information from children about their neighborhoods.

One such study, completed in a middle sized city in the Netherlands, queried children about the places they liked and disliked in their neighborhoods (van Andel, 1990). The sample consisted of 140 children between the ages of 6 and 12 who lived in three different neighborhoods. The three neighborhoods are described in terms of physical layout, but not in terms of socioeconomic or demographic information. Children were asked about places they thought were attractive, boring, and dangerous.

Children in all three of the neighborhoods were most likely to mention places they found attractive. These places tended to include parks or other natural or green areas. The propensity for children to note places such as these coincided with whether or not such areas existed within the neighborhoods. The reasons that children gave for liking any specific area within a neighborhood were that it allowed them to (1) participate in some activity, such as riding bikes or playing soccer, (2) have access to natural items such as trees or simply wide open space, and (3) be in the company of other children (van Andel, 1990).

Children in this study were less likely to note boring areas within their neighborhoods, however, nearly half of the areas labeled boring were playgrounds and streets. The reasons that children gave for the boring nature of these areas were: (1) too much traffic, (2) obstacles that prevented them from playing, (3) litter or other messes, and (4) other children who were mean. As for places children viewed as dangerous, the street was most often mentioned. The danger in the streets was noted to be due to the quantity of cars and the speed at which they traveled. Children noted the potential for being involved in an accident due to the vehicles in the street. This sense of danger is dramatically different from the depictions in the children's drawings noted in Lewis and Osofsky's (1997) study of children in low-income neighborhoods in the United States.

Another study in which children were queried about their neighborhoods was conducted by Schiavo (1988) who worked with 59 children between the ages of 8 and 18 who attended public schools and resided in a middle class suburban area about 15 miles from Boston, Massachusetts. Children were asked to evaluate their neighborhoods in terms of its characteristics and the activities that took place in it. In addition, children were given a camera and instructed to take up to 24 photographs of "any place in the home or neighborhood that's important to you, any place you care about" (Schiavo, 1988, 5). While the children photographed people, animals, and physical places, the author reports on only the photos that involved physical places.

Similar to the children in van Andel's (1990) study, these children favored places that provided opportunities for: (1) activities such as bike riding or playing and (2) positive social relationships with "friends and/ or among neighbors" (Schiavo, 1988, 5). The characteristics children disliked within the neighborhood were busy streets, yard sizes, or the absence of children within their age group. In contrast, the main features of the neighborhood that participants felt were positive for adolescents were their proximity to "highways to get to movies and shopping areas" (Schiavo, 1988, 5). It is notable that as the participants reached older adolescence they became "less place-dependent" or mentioned diminished linkages to the neighborhood of residence for activities and social relations. Instead, they were more aligned with "neighborhoods of sociability" or "places" where they spent time among peers. Schiavo's (1988) study suggests that photographs may be a viable tool for assessment of a child's neighborhood. However, if one is working with adolescents, it may be important to assess neighborhoods of residence as well as neighborhoods of sociability. Another form of research in which children talk about their residential locations results in more open-ended depictions of neighborhood environments. I turn to these next.

Moore (1986) worked with children in the London (U.K.) area to learn about "their specific interactions with their surroundings . . . [her] starting point in understanding the relationship between play, place, and child development, was to find out what children actually did, where, when, with what, with whom—when not in class or at home engaged in routine chores" (Moore, 1986, xvii). The participants in the study were 96 children ages 9 to 12 who lived in three different "city" neighborhoods. All of the children completed a drawing in response to the request to draw a "map or drawing of all of your favorite places–where you go after school or at weekends, including summer–around your home, in the neighbourhood where you live" (Moore, 1986, 268). Each child also participated in a 15 to 20 minute interview. In addition, about one quarter of the children participated in "field trips" in which they acted as experts who took the researcher on a trip around the territory of their neighborhoods (Moore, 1986). Similar to the other studies, attraction and danger are evident in child descriptions of their neighborhoods. Moore's (1986) study suggests that direct social work practitioners who provide home-based services could engage children in a "neighborhood field trip" as part of the assessment process. Bryant (1985) provides an instrument for conducting this type of assessment.

The next study reviewed represents another view of neighborhood from the child's perspective. Burton and Price-Spratlen (1999) report data from a 5-year ethnographic study conducted in a northeastern (USA) city where they learned about "community and family beliefs concerning the definitions of neighborhood, neighborhood processes, and the life-course development of urban African American children, teens, and adults" (p. 83). They note the differences between adult and child definitions of neighborhood boundaries. In fact, in 56% of the cases in their study the children and adolescents defined the boundaries of the neighborhood in a manner that greatly contrasted with the boundaries noted by the adults. One 8-year-old boy said, "Well, my neighborhood is where my best friends live. Eric lives on the corner of Anderson,

Devon lives in the middle of the block on Tyree Street, and Jason lives at the end of the street on Beacon . . . my neighborhood doesn't go past those streets either way. That's my neighborhood" (Burton & Price-Spratlen, 1999, 85). In contrast, this child's mother defined the boundaries of his (the child's) neighborhood to include an area of 5 blocks in one direction and 8 blocks in another because it represented the parameters within which the child could travel safely on foot without her (Burton & Price-Spratlen, 1999).

Another child, an 11-year-old boy, provides an example of the multiple neighborhoods a child may need to negotiate. He states, "Lady, I think you're pretty smart, so let me tell you how it is. When I go to my momma's I have to be a bad ass or I will get beat up. So if you see me over there, I look like that. But when I'm with Nana (grandmother) I'm another way 'cause the kids over there don't fight that much so I don't have to swell-up (act like he's tough) . . ." (Burton & Price-Spratlen, 1999, 87).

Finally, a 12-year-old boy in their sample suggests the way in which the neighborhood can influence residents and vice versa. He says, "My neighborhood so bad is cause some of the young bloods here is bad. Just cause it's all junky round here don't mean people in it got to be junky on the inside. If young brothers round here get together, we could make it a good place. Some my friends don't know that it be bad here cause they be bad not cause the neighborhood make them bad" (Burton & Price-Spratlen, 1999, 88). The findings from this study suggest that (1) the child's voice is a key element in assessing neighborhood, (2) children may be influenced by more than one neighborhood environment, and (3) children do perceive potential linkages between neighborhood conditions and human behavior.

In summary, the literature reviewed here suggests some possible strategies (drawings, verbal reports, photographs, and neighborhood field trips) for assessing the construct "neighborhood." It also illuminates the variety of experiences that occur for children within their neighborhoods of residence. However, while these studies supply a picture of the neighborhood from the child's eye view, they have not been conducted from a social work practice perspective. Thus, they are not instructive for assessments in direct social work practice because they do not demonstrate the actual components that should be included in assessments of the child-neighborhood relationship. In addition, they lack a clear picture of the potential role played by neighbors in children's neighborhood experiences. The study and results presented in the final part of this article contribute toward filling this gap.

STUDY PURPOSE AND QUESTIONS

The study reported here is part of a larger research study aimed at shedding light on the complexity involved in measuring the construct neighborhood. This larger study utilizes a mixed methods approach to explore the intersection and divergence between a traditional quantitative measure of neighborhood based in 2000 census data and a qualitative measure of neighborhood based on the voices of children. For the purposes of this article, the qualitative data are reported as a means to respond to the query: "How can the strength-based lens and practice-orientation of social work be applied in research to enhance our understanding of the construct 'neighborhood' and how can that knowledge be employed to benefit the children we serve?" Therefore, this research explores these questions: (1) How do children describe and interact with the human, natural, and institutional resources in their neighborhoods? (2) What implications do the results hold for assessing the construct "neighborhood" in direct social work practice with children?

METHOD

Participants

The non-random, convenience sample of fourth and fifth grade public school students (N = 59) consists of a diverse group of boys (48%) and girls (52%) representing Euro-Americans (42.2%), Asians and Pacific Islanders (18.6%), Native Americans (15.3%), Mexican Americans (8.5%), Hispanic children of color (6.8%), African Americans (5.1%), Hispanic Whites (1.7%), and Africans (1.7%). A total of 66 children were invited to participate in the study. Four children did not receive permission from their parents to participate in the study. Three children who did have parental permission to participate in the study declined to be respondents. The resulting sample consists of 59 children.

The fourth and fifth grade age group was selected to ensure that the participants were at an age where they are allowed some measure of freedom to explore their neighborhoods. Additionally, at this age children have developed the social and cognitive capacity to respond to the research questions and activities. Also, children in the fourth and fifth grades are learning about maps, neighborhoods, and neighbors. Hence, this project coincides well with their regular curriculum and can benefit their current learning activities.

There are limitations associated with the use of non-random, convenience samples such as the one utilized in this study. For example, access to a sampling frame of all of the fourth and fifth grade classrooms in the district from which a random sample of classrooms could be drawn would have provided for a greater opportunity to generalize from the results to the broader population. However, the fact that the district where the participants attend school operates under "school choice" (i.e., parents can arrange to have their child attend a particular public school even if it is not the school closest to their home) means that there is potential for more diversity within a single classroom than if the children attended schools based solely on their neighborhoods. In fact, the racial demographics of the sample indicate that it is fairly diverse. While there are limitations to the sample, on the whole it does represent a fairly diverse group of children who reside in a fairly diverse group of census tracts that are comparable to the other tracts in the surrounding city. Additionally, the reader will note that elements of the results are comparable to the findings of other studies in which children "speak" about neighborhoods.

The schools and classrooms were selected by virtue of the investigator's connections within the community. Administrators at each school discussed the research study with fourth/fifth grade teachers and one teacher from each school volunteered to work with the investigator. The sample was nearly equally divided between the three different schools. These schools are located in three distinct neighborhood areas within or near an urban environment. Each school represents distinct socio-demographic characteristics. One has a population of students who are predominantly White, lower-middle-class to middle-class. The second school serves a broad range of students from lower to upper socioeconomic groups who are American Indian, African American, and White. The third school serves a mix of students including lower and middle socioeconomic groups, Asian, White, and African American students, including numerous recent immigrants.

The fifty-nine participants represent 30 census tracts within the greater city area. The census variables for these tracts, as measured by 2000 census data, are similar to those of the 136 tracts that constitute the surrounding city area. These similarities in reference to means and standard deviations are noted in Table 1.

Measures

The data were derived from children's written work in response to pre-designed open-ended questions about their neighborhoods and neighbors. This type of approach is similar to other research studies that explore children's relationships to neighborhood environments (Burton & Price-Spratlen, 1999; Figueira-McDonough, 1998; Hart, 1979; Ladd, 1970; Maurer & Baxter, 1972; Sutton, 1992). The questions utilized in the measures are listed in Table 2.

While some scholars discourage the use of pre-designed, structured questions for the collection of qualitative data (Lincoln & Guba, 1985), others suggest a more balanced approach to this decision. Miles and Huberman (1994) note that pre-designed questions are useful in qualita-

TABLE 1. Participant Census Tract Characteristics Compared to Those in the Surrounding City

Census variable, mean, standard deviation	Census variable, mean, standard deviation
% families with incomes $75,000 or more Mean (N = 136/n = 30) 36.6/ 35.8 Standard Dev. (N = 136/n = 30) 16.9/ 20.3	% of population below poverty line Mean (N = 136/n = 30) 12.5/ 12.8 Standard Dev. (N = 136/n = 30) 9.5/ 9.9
% of adults 25 and older with a college education (includes AA to PhD degrees) Mean (N = 136/n = 30) 51.3/ 48.5 Standard Dev. (N = 136/n = 30) 18.6/ 22.3	% households receiving public assistance Mean (N = 136/n = 30) 3.3/ 3.9 Standard Dev. (N = 136/n = 30) 3.4/ 4.0
% of those 16 and older employed in managerial or professional positions Mean (N = 136/n = 30) 46.0/ 44.3 Standard Dev. (N = 136/n = 30) 14.5/ 18.5	% 16 and older who are unemployed Mean (N = 136/n = 30) 3.7/ 3.8 Standard Dev. (N = 136/n = 30) 2.0/ 1.8
% foreign born Mean (N = 136/n = 30) 17.1/ 18.6 Standard Dev. (N = 136/n = 30) 11.0/ 13.4	% female headed families with children 18 years or younger Mean (N = 136/n = 30) 9.7/ 11.0 Standard Dev. (N = 136/n = 30) 6.6/ 8.14
% foreign born who entered the U.S. 1995 to 2000 Mean (N = 136/n = 30) 25.9/ 27.9 Standard Dev. (N = 136/n = 30) 11.4/ 11.3	% 5 years and older living in the same house in 1995 Mean (N = 136/n = 30) 44.0/ 46.5 Standard Dev. (N = 136/n = 30) 13.1/ 12.4

TABLE 2. Question Stems Utilized in Data Collection Measures

Pre-designed question stems	Pre-designed question stems
A place I like in my neighborhood is . . . I like it because . . .	A place I do not like in my neighborhood is . . . I do not like it because . . .
A neighbor I like is . . . I like this neighbor because . . . Some of the things this neighbor does are . . .	Dear . . . These are some of the things I have learned from you . . . These are some of the ways you have helped me . . .

tive data collection when the researcher: (1) knows what he/she is after, (2) wants to ensure a particular focus in order to avoid the collection of "too much superfluous information," (3) wants to create a research project that allows for results that can be compared across studies, (4) has many cases in the sample, and (5) is using multi-methods (i.e., both qualitative and quantitative). These conditions apply to both this study and the larger, mixed methods study from which it is drawn.

In addition, gathering data from children across several large group settings (e.g., classrooms in different schools) requires a degree of uniformity so as to have data that are comparable across the settings and among the large number of children in the sample. The use of pre-designed questions for the data collection in this study was also the most useful way to collect information within the constraints of the classroom setting and amount of time allotted for each data collection session. In fact, Miles and Huberman (1994) note that "Not thinking in instrument design terms (e.g., use of pre-designed questions) can, in fact, lead to self-delusion: You feel 'sensitive' to the site but actually may be stuck in reactive, seat-of-the-pants interviewing" (p. 38). Anyone who has spent time working with classrooms of more than twenty children can imagine the kind of "seat-of-the-pants" interview that could take place in the absence of some pre-designed structure and questions. In essence, the pre-designed structure is what allowed the children in this sample to respond as freely as possible within the classroom setting.

Procedures

The qualitative data were collected late in the spring semester of 2001. All data collection occurred in the classroom setting with children working as individuals to complete writing assignments. The procedures for this study were conducted during four, 45-60 minute periods that took place over a two- to three-week time period that was scheduled at the convenience of each cooperating teacher. Each teacher was present while the investigator conducted the research activities.

Data collection occurred in the form of structured classroom activities that involved discussion and writing. The questions for the individual writing tasks, as previously noted, were open-ended and posed as stems so that the children could rely on some structure, but also have opportunities to respond from their own perspectives. This format was especially useful for this age group as a means to avoid overwhelming them with a full blank page on which to write while at the same time offering the opportunity to respond with their own words. The children indicated their own sense of freedom with these stems in that some noted, "there is no place I like in my neighborhood," or asked if they could write about their mother or father as neighbors because they did not know any neighbors. Naturally, the answer to questions such as these was yes. All of the responses, whether directly to the questions or tailored to individual needs, provided important information about each child's neighborhood experiences.

The investigator and each teacher worked together to reduce the "right answer syndrome" and to encourage original responses by telling the children that these activities were different than what they usually do in school because there are no right or wrong answers. Given the nature of schooling, this reminder occurred regularly and was emphasized by the investigator as she told the children that they are the experts on their neighborhoods.

Data Analysis

Qualitative analysis of written and oral responses has been employed as a means for comprehending how people, especially children, view their neighborhoods (Burton & Price-Spratlen, 1999; Figueira- McDonough, 1998; Hart, 1979; Ladd, 1970; Maurer & Baxter, 1972; Sutton, 1992). While there is a diversity of racial and ethnic groups represented in the sample, the numbers within these categories are quite small to be sufficient for separate analysis. Therefore, the analysis was completed on the data as a whole via the software package ATLAS/ti (Muhr, 1997). This package does not "do" or "think through" the analysis for the researcher; instead it provides a system that allows the researcher to manage the qualitative data analysis.

The constant comparative method of analysis (Lincoln & Guba, 1985) was employed because it allows for the exploration and discovery of subjective experiences and knowledge. It is employed in this data analysis because it leads to "a particular construction of the situation at hand" (Lincoln & Guba, 1985, 343) which in this case refers to the children's reports or constructions of their actual neighborhood experiences. This emphasis on understanding the children's construction of their neighborhoods (i.e., the situation at hand) differs from the goal of grounded theory analysis as conceptualized by Glaser and Strauss (1967) and Strauss and Corbin (1998). In other words, when the constant comparative method is utilized in the tradition of Glaser and Strauss (1967) and Strauss and Corbin (1998), the major goal is the production of a grounded theory. Given that this research is exploratory in nature and does not aspire to create a grounded theory or to test theory, it was most useful to follow the constant comparative analysis process as outlined by Lincoln and Guba (1985).

Limitations

The limitations of any research can be summed up in terms of issues of validity and reliability. This is true for the study at hand even though it is exploratory in nature and does not predict outcome variables. Conceptualizations of validity and reliability differ between quantitative and qualitative research (Franklin & Ballan, 2001; Lincoln & Guba, 1985; Stauss & Corbin, 1998). The issues of validity and reliability will be addressed within the qualitative conceptual framework that employs the concepts of credibility, transferability, and dependability (Franklin & Ballan, 2001; Lincoln & Guba, 1985; Guba & Lincoln, 1989).

Miles (1979) notes that the "most serious and central difficulty in the use of qualitative data is that the methods of analysis are not well formulated" (p. 591). Given this, special care was taken to follow the guidelines specified by Lincoln and Guba (1985) for employing the constant comparative method of analysis (see Nicotera, 2003 for detailed descriptions of the development of codes and categories under the auspices of this method). The constant comparative analysis allowed the emerging codes and categories to remain close to the empirical data (Franklin & Ballan, 2001) or kept the researcher grounded in the data (Glaser & Strauss, 1967). This closeness to the data is evidenced in the use of local language found in the codes and categories as well as the manner in which direct quotes from the data support the categories or dimensions of neighborhood. Additionally, every measure was taken to ensure that the voices of the children would be heard in the study results. For example, it would have been easy for the researcher to list "church" as a formal resource in the category that describes the resources in the neighborhoods even though a child noted that it was something she/he disliked. Hence, while an adult may view "church" as a resource for a child whether or not the child likes it, it was important to let the child's voice to be heard by only including items as a resource, for example, when a child noted them as a positive attribute in her or his neighborhood experiences. Another technique for considering the emerging codes and categories involved the participation of three colleagues who reviewed codes and quotations and assisted in final decisions about the face validity of the codes, categories, and original quotations. This process was extremely useful in finalizing the categories and subcategories as they emerged from the data.

The features noted above provide for credibility, transferability, and dependability as described by Franklin and Ballan (2001) and Lincoln and Guba (1985). Furthermore, the use of the computer program, ATLAS/ti (Muhr, 1997) provided consistency in how the data were handled which is recommended by Franklin and Ballan (2001) as a means to account for credibility. Finally, the issue of dependability, which is specifically related to issues of replication, is addressed within this study in several ways. While this study has not yet been replicated, the use of pre-designed questions, clear parameters of the sample demographics of the children and census tracks, and the specific use of the constant comparative method (Lincoln & Guba, 1985) create a foundation for the replication of this study. Worth mentioning is that some of the findings from this study, in terms of how children describe their neighborhoods of residence, are comparable to the findings of other studies that were outlined in the literature review. Additionally, the sample size ($N = 59$) of this study exceeds the recommended number of cases (8 to 15) for "establishing consistency in findings and providing examples to initially hypothesize about the limits of those findings" (Hill, Thompson, & Williams, 1997 as cited in Franklin & Ballan, 2001, p. 278).

RESULTS

Nine dimensions (37 sub-dimensions) of the construct "neighborhood" emerged from the analysis of the children's narratives. These dimensions represent places and neighbors that provide opportunities for children to attain competencies that range from cognitive and physical skills to social-emotional skills and capacities for nurturing of others, as well as for independence. In addition, the dimensions indicate that the children in this sample receive both tangible and intangible supports from their neighbors and that they have access to resources within the natural and built environment to support their development. Problems are also identified in reference to the absence of adequate play spaces and playmates and the presence of unsavory characters, as well in relation to some of the neighborhood related emotions experienced by study participants. The dimensions, their respective sub-dimensions, and code examples are noted in Figures 1 through 5.

I differentiate among the nine dimensions in terms of their relevance to the assessment of the child-neighborhood relationship in direct social work practice as compared to their relevance to measuring the construct neighborhood within the context of social welfare research. All nine dimensions are clearly relevant within social welfare research that endeavors to create a more comprehensive measure for the construct neighborhood. However, five of the dimensions demonstrate elements of the child-neighborhood relationship that are most pertinent for assessing this construct within the context of *direct* social work practice. In addition, these five are also *clearly significant* in measuring the construct neighborhood within the context of social welfare research. However, the four other dimensions, the people I know, the people in my neighborhood, the built environment, and the natural environment, are not examined in this article because they do not provide the social work practitioner with any further information that is relevant for the direct practice assessment of the child-neighborhood relationship. Consider the following two examples: (1) the dimension, "the people in my neighborhood" contains codes and sub-dimensions that represent the listing of people that emerged from the children's responses (e.g., homeless people, the neighbor across the street, good friends, drunks), and (2) the two dimensions the "built and natural environments" provide lists about what the child sees within her or his neighborhood (e.g., a church, a field, a library). The reader will see, as this section of the article unfolds, that these more skeletal or bare bones components of the construct neighborhood, as described in the two examples above, come alive in the other five dimensions that are deemed as more pertinent to direct practice assessments. For example, the "built and natural environments" come to life in the dimension "resources" which exposes the children's subjective renderings of the built and natural elements of the neighborhood that they viewed as desirable. In addition, the dimension "the people in my neighborhood," expands beyond a mere list within the dimensions "the feel of the neighborhood," "support," and "competence."

In summary, the inclusion of all nine of the dimensions within social welfare research remains important as a means for gaining a fuller comprehension of how to measure the construct neighborhood from both an objective and subjective perspective. However, direct practice social work assessments seek to gain understanding of the more subjective experiences that create clients' unique understandings of themselves and the world around them. Therefore, I have limited the discussion to the five dimensions presented in this section. I begin this discussion next.

The dimension "competence" emerged from data and codes that noted the child had learned something via social interaction with neighbors. This category *excludes* other activities through which the children had opportunities to develop competence (e.g., going to the store to buy chips and pop) because activities such as this were not noted to have coincided with the guidance of a neighbor. Thus, the key to the category competence is that competence was gained via social interaction or experiences with an identified neighbor. It was the active nature of teaching or assisting toward competence, as identified by the children that allowed a code to be included in this category. These experiences, of gaining competence under the tutelage of a neighbor were further divided into the eight sub-dimensions. This dimension, the eight sub-dimensions, and code examples are displayed in Figure 1. The dimension is noted in the center of the figure with the sub-dimensions and related code examples radiating out from that center circle. This type of display is repeated for all of the dimensions, sub-dimensions, and code examples displayed in this section.

Adults view competence and mastery as key developmental tasks for middle childhood. Interestingly, the social interactions that are salient

FIGURE 1. The Dimension Competence, Its Sub-Dimensions, Code Examples

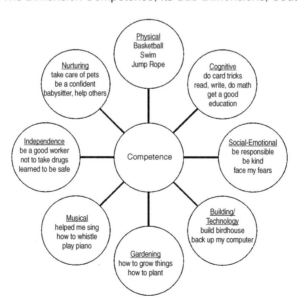

for the children in this sample mirror this major component associated with their developmental phase. The connection between these social interactions and competency becomes evident in the following quotes. For example, this quote demonstrates that the child practiced social emotional, cognitive, and physical skills in relation to a neighbor. "Dear Mr. B., These are some of the things I have learned from you. (1) If you give someone something they will give me something back, (2) you should be nice, (3) how to walk and read at the same time." The next quote indicates that the child gained competence in social-emotional skills and building and technology skills: "Dear J., These are some of the things I have learned from you. You have taught me to face my fears, you taught me to blow bubbles, and you taught me how to install things on the internet." Another child notes practice of skills for independence, social-emotional capacity, and building and technology. "Dear S., You have taught me how to be a gentleman. And you have taught me manners. You have taught me how to use a computer and how to play games. You have also taught me how to save money and put it in a safe place." The next quote notes competence for gardening and nurturing. "These are some of the ways you have helped me. You have helped me in so many ways like how to feed a cat and how to plant a plant."

It is important to note here that the children in this sample do not always use the term "neighbor" in the traditional sense of neighbor as a non-related person. As noted previously, some of the children chose to write about a family member as a neighbor because they either did not know a neighbor or could not think of one at that moment in time. While some children (n = 18) noted that the "neighbor" who taught them was a family member, the majority of the children (n = 35) wrote about learning from a neighbor who was not a member of their family. Six of the children noted that the "neighbor" they learned from is their current teacher, even though, they do not live in the same neighborhood as that teacher. Thus, while family and teachers show up as important for the development of competence, non-related neighbors have a large presence in this dimension of the construct neighborhood. The next dimension, "support," also involves neighbors as important players in the lives of the participants.

The dimension "support" (see Figure 2) represents codes from the data that described instances of neighboring that provided some tangible support such as a neighbor babysitting a child or taking a child to the library. The data also presented instances of intangible support such as cheering a child up when he or she was down and giving advice for

FIGURE 2. The Dimension Support, Its Sub-Dimensions, Code Examples

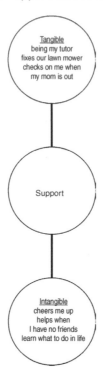

when a child grows up. While competence involves the teaching of skills, support involves being available for a child (and his or her family) in either a hands-on manner (e.g., the neighbor who mows a child's lawn) or a more subtle way that provides, for instance, emotional support (e.g., the neighbor who helps a child when he or she has no friends).

The elements of support mentioned by the children are not dissimilar from the elements of support that adults might look for in their own day-to-day social interactions. The following examples represent the reception of both tangible and intangible support. "I like this neighbor because she is nice to me and when I get locked out she lets me go inside her house. And she lets me eat in her house." "He helps me have fun when I'm bored. He cheers me up. He babysits." "You cheered me up when I cry and you helped me make dough and you cooked the dough so good it tasted like cherry." "She gave me and my friend lollipops once.

I like this neighbor because she is always happy to see us and smiles and waves at us." It is important to mention that not all participants noted both types of support and a small number did not note the reception of any support. The next dimension reported, "the feel of the neighborhood," is less about social interaction and more about the sentiments that emerged from what the children wrote in response to the study measures.

While most of the quotes that characterize the dimensions discussed thus far are positive, the next dimension, "the feel of the neighborhood" (see Figure 3), provides some of the more negative characteristics of the

FIGURE 3. The Dimension, the Feel of the Neighborhood, Its Sub-Dimensions, Code Examples

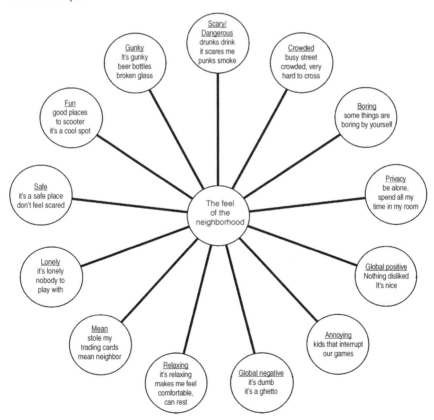

neighborhoods in which the participants reside. In fact, the majority of the sub-dimensions reflect negative emotions.

The dimension of neighborhood noted in Figure 3 emerged from codes that reflected some emotion about the neighborhood. For example, the sub-dimension "scary/dangerous" mirrors the use of that word, by the children, to describe some aspect of the neighborhood. For example, one participant wrote, "A place I do not like in my neighborhood is Broadway at night. I do not like it because it is dangerous." Another participant noted the following in reference to a bar: "I do not like it because dumb, stupid, drunkies get drink there."

On a lighter note, some of the participants expressed more positive sentiments about their neighborhoods. For example, one child wrote this about the library: "I like it because it's quiet and I like to read." Another child wrote this about the fire station: "I like the fire station just because I have self-confidence in them." Still a third child noted feeling safe: "I like it because it makes me feel safe and comfortable that I am in my own place and someone is there." The last two dimensions reported here, "activity" and "resources," are related more to the physical neighborhood environment, though they clearly encompass the participants' subjective experiences.

Codes and quotes were included in the "activity" dimension (see Figure 4) if they described some action the child took within the neighborhood. The activities were easily placed in the four sub-dimensions

FIGURE 4. The Dimension Activities, Its Sub-Dimensions, Code Examples

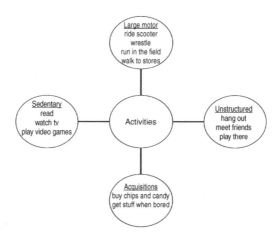

displayed in Figure 4. For example, some children described activities that involved large motor skills (e.g., riding a bike). These were easily differentiated from descriptions of activities that do not usually require use of large motor skills such as reading or watching TV (sedentary) or activities that involved buying chips at the store (acquisitions).

Quotes that represent the two sub-dimensions, sedentary and large motor activities are: "I like my room because I can watch TV and play my play station" and "I like it because it has a little field. You can run around and play with your dog." Quotes that represent "acquisitions" include: "Sometimes my friend T. and I go to the volleyball court. We go to the store to buy chips or candy" and "I like it because you can get cool things there when you're hungry, thirsty, or bored."

Perhaps the most subtle sub-dimension in the activity dimension is "unstructured," which includes any mention of undefined or minimally defined "hanging out" or "playing." Quotes that portray this sub-dimension are: "I like the parks that are in my neighborhood because I could spend time with my family" and "I like it because I and my friend hang out at my tree house."

The last dimension reported here is labeled, "resources" and has some overlap with the "activity" dimension because the option for participants to engage in some activities was often linked to the existence of a neighborhood resource. The sub-dimensions and related codes for the "resource" dimension are displayed in Figure 5.

FIGURE 5. The Dimension Resources, Its Sub-Dimensions, Code Examples

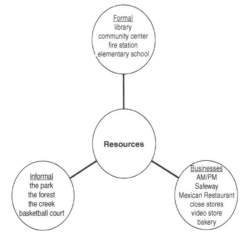

The codes and quotes that make up the dimension "resources" represent entities in the neighborhood that the children note liking or using for their benefit. For example, one child wrote about the forest, "A place I like in my neighborhood is the forest right next to my house. I like it because I like building club houses with sticks and branches." The forest then became an informal resource (not connected to a formal social organization) within the child's neighborhood. If a child wrote about something in the neighborhood, but disliked it, then that entity was not included in the resource dimension. For example, one child wrote, "A place I do not like in my neighborhood is the park. I do not like it because it is in the woods and no one really goes there." Hence, this was coded the "park not liked" and *not* included in the list of resources because, as far as the child is concerned, the park is not a resource, even though any passerby might see the park and consider it a neighborhood resource.

Another example of this contradiction within the resources dimension emerges from the sub-dimension "businesses." One child wrote about the 7/11 store in the neighborhood, "A place I do not like in my neighborhood is the Seven Eleven across from the fire station. I do not like it because it attracts drunks, smokers, and people who sell drugs." Thus, this would not be viewed, by this child, as a resource and it was not included in the resource dimension. However, another child wrote, "A place I like in my neighborhood is the 7/11 and the Safeway." Therefore, the "7/11 liked" was noted, in this case, as a resource.

There is a similar contradiction within the "formal resource" sub-dimension in which one child wrote about liking church and another wrote about disliking it. The codes and quotes that make up this sub-dimension entered it because they referred to some neighborhood entity a child liked or used in a beneficial way and were connected to a formal organization, such as church, a community center or a school. A point of distinction must be made here. There were some resources such as football fields, swimming pools, and basketball courts that may actually be connected to some formal organization such as a school or community center. However, unless the child referenced such a resource as being at the community center or school, I did not feel I should impose my assumption about this on the data and therefore these entities are noted as informal resources.

DISCUSSION

The purpose of this study was to explore how the strength-based lens and practice orientation of social work can be applied in research to enhance our understanding of the construct "neighborhood" and how that knowledge can be employed to benefit the children we serve. Two questions were posed for this exploration: (1) How do children describe and interact with the human, natural, and institutional resources in their neighborhoods? (2) What implications do the results hold for assessing the construct "neighborhood" in direct social work practice with children? The findings are discussed in light of these questions.

In summary, the results represent a myriad of children's positive and negative neighborhood descriptions of and interactions with the human, natural, and institutional resources within the locales where they reside. The themes that emerge from the data encompass the following: neighbors, emotions, physicality, activity, support, and learning. The findings indicate that the ways in which the children describe and interact with their neighborhoods are interrelated. For example, a description of a park or a house involves how it is used or what is seen there. Descriptions of people also encompass the roles they play in how children use and experience the neighborhood environment. Additionally, the descriptions of neighborhood that reveal emotions also reflect certain activities that occur or do not occur. Hence, these data indicate the overlap between the conception of neighborhood as a physical entity and neighborhood as composed of social processes and subjective experiences. These three elements, physicality, social processes, and subjectivity, were discussed earlier in this article as important components in comprehending the construct "neighborhood." The second aim of this study is to apply the results to illuminate a means for conducting direct practice social work assessments of the child-neighborhood relationship. A discussion of the results and their implications for such assessments follows.

This research demonstrates that when viewed through the lens of the children who reside within them, neighborhood environments do have the capacity to enrich as well as the potential to undermine their lives. It suggests that direct social work practitioners add "neighborhood" as an important element in bio-psycho-social assessments of children in order to gain a picture of the ways in which it positively and/or negatively influences them. Accounting for the strengths *and* challenges of a child's neighborhood has the potential to enhance social work interventions. For example, a child's neighborhood activities and/or relationships may represent capacities in a child who might have an otherwise difficult life within her/his family or school. When viewed through the eyes of a child client, the practitioner may discover that the neighborhood serves as a site for previously unidentified social support. Or, the social worker may learn about neighborhood-based activities in which the child engages that support important skills, such as the ability to plan and use unstructured time, or the development of positive peer relationships.

On the other hand, assessing the child-neighborhood relationship may uncover significant problems for a child that can be addressed within the context of the helping relationship. For example, if a child notes scary/dangerous feelings about some aspect of his or her neighborhood, such as the drug dealers on the corner, the social worker then has the opportunity to facilitate a family discussion about the feelings. Such discussions can be useful in helping a child to resist incorporating these elements into her or his self-identity. Similarly, a child who points out that broken bottles and trash create hazardous play areas provides an opportunity for his or her family and the social worker to discuss ways in which neighborhood residents can be empowered to have those play areas cleaned up. Given the utility of including the neighborhood environment in social work assessments with children, I turn now to a discussion of how these results inform the development of tools for the assessment of child-neighborhood relationships.

The results specify four key components to include in direct practice assessments of child-neighborhood relationships. These components are:

1. the child's identification of social processes with neighbors who assist in the development of competence and provide support,
2. the child's sentiments (positive and negative) about the people and places within the neighborhood,
3. the neighborhood-based activities in which the child engages,
4. the child identified resources available within the neighborhood.

Obtaining assessment data about both the positive and negative aspects of these components is paramount. This requires social workers to listen for what is "said" as well as what is "not said" by a child during the neighborhood assessment phase. For example, if a practitioner is posing an open-ended question related to neighborhood-based activities (component 3) and a child has no response or reports only activities outside of the neighborhood, then the practitioner will want to inquire further about what may be missing from the neighborhood.

While social workers who are interested in the inclusion of child-neighborhood relationship assessments are encouraged to employ the four components to create their own open-ended assessment questions, the outcome of this research suggests that detailed information about the positive and negative aspects of the child-neighborhood relationship can be gained successfully by utilizing the opened-ended question stems noted previously in Table 2. For example, asking the children in this sample what they like and do not like about their neighborhoods produced a mix of positive and negative sentiments about the conditions of the neighborhoods where they reside. Additionally, the cultural and gender diversity represented in this sample suggests that these question stems could be utilized successfully with both boys and girls as well as with children from varying cultural backgrounds. While the data collection for this study employed written responses to these question stems, in social work practice the form of response could be oral or drawn as well as written, depending on the needs of the child.

The incorporation of neighborhood as a component of the bio-psycho-social assessment could occur at the level of individual practitioners, or social work agencies may choose to add neighborhood as an element for inclusion on intake forms. Whether the element neighborhood is assessed at the discretion of individual practitioners or formalized as part of agency intake forms, some training is indicated. For example, as with any social work assessment procedure, self-awareness is an important ingredient. Therefore, it would be important for training to encourage social workers to discover and be mindful of the assumptions they may hold about the neighborhoods where their child clients reside. These assumptions may serve as obstacles to a practitioner's capacity to see strengths in some neighborhoods as well as to see challenges in others. In addition, assessment data gathered from exploring the child-neighborhood relationship may indicate a need for intervention that goes beyond the direct practice relationship. Consequently, any training on the inclusion of neighborhood as part of the bio-psycho-social assessment process should also include frameworks for enlisting the cooperation of community-oriented social workers who could conduct macro assessments and interventions, if warranted.

Finally, social work educators are in a position to educate students to view neighborhood as an integral part of bio-psycho-social assessments. At this juncture, given the dearth of social work-oriented research on neighborhoods, this would require an interdisciplinary orientation toward assigned readings, some of which are referenced in this article. In conjunction with readings, social work students will benefit from field-related assignments that introduce them to child-neighborhood assessments and interventions at both the micro and macro level.

In conclusion, this study demonstrates that lending a strength-based and practice orientation to research on neighborhoods is an endeavor that provides evidence for a more holistic approach to social work assessments with children. The findings indicate four components that are integral to assessing child-neighborhood relationships. In addition, the measures employed in the data collection represent a means for successfully completing such assessments. It is my hope that future neighborhood-oriented research will continue this type of exploration.

REFERENCES

Brodsky, A. (1996). Resilient single mothers in risky neighborhoods: Negative psychological sense of community. *Journal of Community Psychology, 24* (4), 347-363.

Brooks-Gunn, J., Duncan, G., & Aber, J. (1997). *Neighborhood poverty volume one: Context and consequences for children.* New York: Russell Sage Foundation.

Bryant, L. (1985). *The neighborhood walk: Sources of support in middle childhood.* Monographs for the Society of Child development, *50* (3), Serial No. 210.

Burton, L., & Price-Spratlen, T. (1999). Through the eyes of children: An ethnographic perspective on neighborhoods and child development. In A. S. Hasten (Ed.), *Cultural processes in child development* (pp. 77-96). Mahwah, NJ: Lawrence Erlbaum Associates.

Coulton, C., Korbin, J., Su, M., & Chow, J. (1995). Community level factors and child maltreatment rates. *Child Development, 66,* 1262-1276.

Crane, J. (1991). The epidemic theory of ghettos and neighborhood effects on dropping out and teenage childbearing. *American Journal of Sociology, 96* (5), 1226-1259.

David, T., & Weinstein, C. (1987). The built environment and children's development. In Carol Weinstein (Ed.), *Spaces for children: The built environment and child development* (pp. 3-20). New York: Plenum Press.

Figueira-McDonough, J. (1998). Environment and interpretation: Voices of young people in poor inner-city neighborhoods. *Youth and Society, 30* (2), 123-163.

Garbarino, J., Galambos, N., Plantz, M., & Kostenly, K. (1992). The territory of childhood. In J. Garbarino (Ed.), *Children and families in the social environment* (2nd. ed.) (pp. 202-229). New York: Aldine de Gruyter, Inc.

Glaser, B., & Strauss, A. (1967). *The discovery of grounded theory: Strategies for qualitative research.* New York: Aldine De Gruyter.

Guba, E., & Lincoln, Y. (1989). *Fourth generation evaluation.* London: Sage Publications.

Halpern, R. (1995). *Rebuilding the inner city: A history of neighborhood initiatives to address poverty in the United States.* New York: Columbia University Press.

Hart, R. (1979). *Children's experiences of place.* New York: Irvington Publishers.

Hill, C., Thompson, B., & Williams, E. (1997). A guide to conducting consensual qualitative research. *The Consulting Psychologist, 25,* 517-527.

Kemp, S., Whittacker, J., & Tracy, E. (1997). *Person-environment practice: The social ecology of interpersonal helping.* New York: Aldine De Gruyter.

Ladd, F. C. (1970). Black youths view their environment: Neighborhood maps. *Environment and Behavior.* June, 74-99.

Lewis, M., & Osofsky, J. (1997). Violent cities, violent streets: Children draw their neighborhoods. In J. Osofsky (Ed.), *Children in a violent society* (pp. 277-299). New York: Guilford Press.

Lincoln, Y., & Guba, E. (1985). *Naturalistic inquiry.* Beverly Hills, CA: Sage Publications.

Lynch, K. (1979). The spatial world of the child. In L. Michelson (Ed.), *The child in the city: Today and tomorrow* (pp. 102-127). Toronto: University of Toronto Press.

Maurer, R., & Baxter, J. (1972). Images of the neighborhood and city among black, Anglo, and Mexican-American children. *Environment and Behavior,* December, 351-388.

Miles, M. (1979). Qualitative data as an attractive nuisance: The problem of analysis. *Administrative Science Quarterly, 24,* 590-601.

Miles, M., & Huberman, A. (1994). *Qualitative data analysis: An expanded sourcebook* (2nd ed.). Thousand Oaks, CA: Sage Publications.

Moore, R. (1986). *Children's domain: Play and place in child development.* London: Croom Helm.

Muhr, T. (1997). *ATLAS/ti* (version 4.1) [computer software]. Berlin: Scientific Software Development.

Nicotera, N. (2003). *Children and their neighborhoods: A mixed methods approach to understanding the construct neighborhood.* Dissertation Abstracts International, *63* (11), 4095A. (UMI No. 3072123).

Perkins, D., Meeks, J., & Taylor, R. (1992). The physical environment of street blocks and residential perceptions of crime and disorder: Implications for theory and measurement. *Journal of Environmental Psychology, 12,* 21-34.

Proshanksy, H., Fabian, A., & Kaminoff, R. (1983). Place-identity: Physical world socialization of the self. *Journal of Environmental Psychology, 3,* 57-83.

Rivlin, L. (1987). The neighborhood, personal identity, and group affiliations. In Altman and Wandersman (Eds.), *Neighborhood and community environment* (pp. 1-34). New York: Plenum Press.

Sampson, R., & Groves, W. (1989). Community structure and crime: Testing social-disorganization theory. *American Journal of Sociology, 94* (4), 774-802.

Schiavo, R. S. (1988). Age differences in assessment and use of a suburban neighborhood among children and adolescents. *Children's Environments Quarterly, 5* (2), 4-9.

Simcha-Fagin, O., & Schwartz, J. (1986). Neighborhood and delinquency: An assessment of contextual effects. *Criminology, 24* (4), 667-704.

Skejaeveland, O., & Garling, T. (1997). Effects of interactional space on neighboring. *Journal of Environmental Psychology, 17,* 181-198.

Strauss, A., & Corbin, J. (1998). *The basics of qualitative research: Techniques and procedures for developing grounded theory* (2nd ed.). London: Sage.

Sutton, S. (1992). Enabling children to map out a more equitable society. *Children's Environments, 9* (1), 37-48.

Sutton, S. (1996). *Weaving a tapestry of resistance: The places, power, and poetry of a sustainable society.* London: Bergin and Garvey.

Taylor, A., Wiley, A., Kuo, F., & Sullivan, W. (1998). Growing up in the inner city green spaces as places to grow. *Environment and Behavior, 30* (1), 3-27.

Tienda, M. (1991). Poor people and poor places: Deciphering neighborhood effects on poverty outcomes. In J. Huber (Ed.), *Macro-micro linkages in sociology* (pp. 244-262). London: Sage Publications.

van Andel, J. (1990). Places children like, dislike, and fear. *Children's Environments Quarterly. 7* (4), 24-31.

Assessment of Depressive Symptomatology in Young Maltreated Children

Alan J. Litrownik

Rae R. Newton

John A. Landsverk

SUMMARY. The present study examined the characteristics of a self-report measure of depression in young maltreated children. Two samples, Foster Care ($N = 197$) and Clinic Referred ($N = 107$), of mal-

Alan J. Litrownik, PhD, is affiliated with the Department of Psychology, San Diego State University. John A. Landsverk, PhD, is affiliated with the School of Social Work, San Diego State University.

Rae R. Newton, PhD, is affiliated with the Department of Sociology, California State University, Fullerton.

Address correspondence to: Alan J. Litrownik, Associate Director, Child and Adolescent Services Research Center, 3020 Children's Way MC 5033, San Diego, CA 92123-4282.

The research reported herein was supported by grants from the National Institute of Mental Health (R01-46078-01) and USDHHS: Administration for Children, Youth, and Families (90CA1458). Additional support was provided by the NIMH Child and Adolescent Services Research Center, Children's Hospital and Health Center, San Diego, CA.

The authors express their appreciation to the children and their caregivers who participated in this study, and to the administrators and staff of the Children's Services Bureau, Department of Social Services, San Diego County, and the Chadwick Center, Children's Hospital and Health Center, San Diego, for their cooperation.

[Haworth co-indexing entry note]: "Assessment of Depressive Symptomatology in Young Maltreated Children." Litrownik, Alan J., Rae R. Newton, and John A. Landsverk. Co-published simultaneously in *Journal of Human Behavior in the Social Environment* (The Haworth Social Work Practice Press, an imprint of The Haworth Press, Inc.) Vol. 11, No. 3/4, 2005, pp. 135-156; and: *Approaches to Measuring Human Behavior in the Social Environment* (ed: William R. Nugent) The Haworth Social Work Practice Press, an imprint of The Haworth Press, Inc., 2005, pp. 135-156. Single or multiple copies of this article are available for a fee from The Haworth Document Delivery Service [1-800-HAWORTH, 9:00 a.m. - 5:00 p.m. (EST). E-mail address: docdelivery@haworthpress.com].

Available online at http://www.haworthpress.com/web/JHBSE
doi:10.1300/J137v11n03_07

treated children between the ages of 3- and 7-years, were administered the Preschool Symptom Self-Report (PRESS). In addition, a subsample of the foster and all of the clinic children between the ages of 4- and 7-years responded to Harter's measure of Perceived Competence and Social Acceptance. Finally, caregivers completed the Child Behavior Checklist. Results indicate (1) good internal consistency of the measure across samples, ethnic groups, gender, and age (alphas = .86-.89), (2) children removed for physical abuse, younger children and girls were more likely to report depressive symptomatology, (3) self-reported depressive symptomatology was inversely related to self-reported competence and acceptance, and (4) external raters were more likely to agree with each other and with self-reported depressive symptomatology in the youngest children. Thus, some support for the reliability and validity of the PRESS was obtained. *[Article copies available for a fee from The Haworth Document Delivery Service: 1-800-HAWORTH. E-mail address: <docdelivery@haworthpress.com> Website: <http://www. HaworthPress.com> © 2005 by The Haworth Press, Inc. All rights reserved.]*

KEYWORDS. Assessment, depression, maltreated children, childhood depression, measuring depression, foster care

There is a growing recognition that school-aged children and adolescents can suffer from depressive disorders, and that these disorders are likely to continue if treatment is not provided (Kovacs & Goldston, 1991). The importance of assessing depressive symptomatology and providing needed interventions is obvious. It is also becoming apparent that assessments of younger children are necessary as depressive disorders can be evidenced in preschoolers (Kashani & Carlson, 1985), and early depressive symptomatology in young children may be predictive of later problems (Blatt & Homann, 1992; Ialongo, Edelsohn, Werthamer-Larsson, Crockett, & Kellam, 1993). Children who have been maltreated are especially at risk for developing depressive symptomatology that may persist (e.g., Allen & Tarnowski, 1989; Cohen, Adler, Kaplan, Pelcovitz, & Mandel, 2002; Kaufman, 1991; Koverola, Pound, Heger, & Lytle, 1993; Manly, Kim, Rogosch, & Cicchetti, 2001; Mannarino, Cohen, Smith, & Moore-Motily, 1991; Okun, Parker, & Levendosky, 1994; Silverman, Reinherz, & Giaconia, 1996).

For example, Koverola et al. (1993) reported that 67% of their population of sexually abused 6- to 12-year-old children were depressed, while Kaufman (1991) found 27% of 56 7- to 12-year-old maltreated children to have a diagnosis of Major Depression or Dysthymia based on the Kiddie-SADS. In addition to the experience of maltreatment, there is some suggestion that out-of-home placement puts children at additional risk for depression (Rosenfeld, Pilowsky, Fine, Thorpe, Fein, Simms, Halfon, Irwin, Alfaro, Saletsky, & Nickman, 1997) with characteristics of the placement (e.g., type, number, duration) moderating the impact.

Attempts to assess depressive symptoms in, or internal states of, children and adolescents have typically involved reports from those in the individual's environment (e.g., parent, teacher). These informants usually focus on external responses, possibly missing much information about the child's or adolescent's feelings. As a result, self-report measures have been developed for school-aged children and adolescents. Though there is a continuing debate about which of the self-report measures or scales provides the best information (e.g., Hodges, Gordon, & Lennon, 1990), the important overarching concern relates to who is the best informant. The lack of correspondence between reports of depressive symptomatology by older children and adolescents, and external informants demonstrates the need to assess directly the child or adolescent (Barrett, Berney, Bhate, Famuyiwa, Fundudis, Kolvin, & Tyrer, 1991; Hodges et al., 1990). This is critical for maltreated children who have been removed from their home, as informants may not know the child well enough to provide reliable reports. Additionally, incentives to under- or even over-report problems may exist for biological parents, foster parents, and relatives. This is likely to be a problem when the respondent believes that her responses will impact child placement decisions (e.g., reunification with the biological parent, adoption, guardianship, and long-term foster care).

Attempts to assess depressive symptomatology in younger children have only recently emerged (Martini, Strayhorn, & Puig-Antich, 1990). The delay in developing self-report measures is due, in part, to the belief by some (e.g., Digdon & Gotlib, 1985) that young children are not developmentally capable of understanding, much less experiencing, the cognitive symptoms that are associated with depressive disorders. On the other hand, the feasibility of such assessments is suggested by reports of measures that have been developed for individuals of limited cognitive abilities (Harter & Pike, 1984; Litrownik & Steinfeld, 1982). Respondents are typically presented with two or more pictures that are associated with various feelings, expectancies, etc. The respondent must first associate the feelings with the picture, and then select the one that "is most like you." Typical validity checks (i.e., evidence that the child can perform the task) include presentation of items that can be evaluated externally such as a picture of a boy and a picture of a girl, and asking "which one is most like you?" Incorrect selections can be followed by some training before another check, or a decision not to continue can be made. In any case, subsequent items assessing internal states are only presented if the external validity check is passed.

Martini et al. (1990) developed such a pictorial scale, the Preschool Symptom Self-Report (PRESS) to assess depressive symptoms. They presented the 25-item PRESS to a population of 84 Head Start Children (3-years, 2-months, to 5-years, 2-months; 94% Anglo, 6% African-American). The children completed the PRESS, parents and teachers responded to an adult informant version of the PRESS, as well as to other standard external informant measures of affect in children (e.g., CBCL, General Rating of Affective Symptoms–GRASP). Martini et al. (1990) report that the scale was reliable, i.e., internally consistent (Cronbach's Alpha Coefficient = 0.89) and constant over time (24-hour test-retest reliability = 0.86). While they found evidence for concurrent validity with the adult informants (Parent PRESS, Parent CBCL, and Parent GRASP r's = 0.54 to 0.68; Parent and Teacher PRESS r = 0.37), child reports on the PRESS were not related to parent or teacher PRESS reports (r's = $-.07$ and $-.20$, respectively). Finally, they reported that the PRESS was not related to intellectual functioning as measured by the Peabody Picture Vocabulary Test–Revised.

The lack of concordance between reports of the children and adults is not surprising. Hodges et al. (1990) reviewed the research assessing parent-child concordance on various structured interviews. They conclude that concordance is poor overall, but especially problematic for internalizing disorders such as anxiety and depression. While this lack of concordance necessarily limits claims for the validity of a measure, Hodges et al. (1990) argue that it does not serve as conclusive evidence for the lack of validity. That is, concordance on measures of internalizing disorders by a targeted individual and an external observer yields information about interinformant agreement. If there is concordance, evidence of validity is obtained, but the failure to find agreement can be due to either differences in the informants (e.g., perceptions, biases, actual experiences) or problems with the measure.

The PRESS is the only self-report measure of depressive symptomatology that has been developed specifically for children under 8 years of age. It should be noted that Ialongo et al. (1993) modified the Children's Depression Inventory (CDI) for use with a population of first grade children, while others (e.g., Rudolph, Hammen, & Burge, 1994) have administered the CDI to children younger than the measure was initially intended to assess (cf. Smucker, Craighead, Craighead, & Green, 1986). While there is clearly a need for such a measure, especially for populations at risk for developing disorders of affect, additional evidence of its usefulness (e.g., psychometric properties, relationship to socio-demographic factors, and interinformant agreement) is required. In an effort to explore further the usefulness of the PRESS, we assessed (1) 197 maltreated children who were placed in out-of-home (i.e., Foster) care, and (2) 107 children referred for treatment because of abuse. The following were examined: (1) Characteristics of the measure, e.g., overall internal consistency, and consistency across ethnic groups, gender, and age, (2) The relationship of sample characteristics (e.g., gender, ethnicity, age, intellectual functioning) to the PRESS scores, (3) Maltreatment experience of the foster care sample (i.e., reason for removal from home) and its relationship to PRESS scores, (4) The relationship between PRESS scores and scores on an established self-report measure (i.e., Harter Pictorial Scale of Perceived Competence and Social Acceptance), and (5) The relationship between PRESS scores and reports from other informants (i.e., caregiver, interviewer/observer).

METHODS

Subjects

Sample 1. The first sample of children who participated in this study was selected from a larger cohort of children and adolescents (ages 0-17) who had entered out-of-home care due to maltreatment between May, 1990 and October, 1991 in San Diego County and remained in placement for at least 5 months ($N = 1,221$). Children between 3- and 7-years of age were included in the present study. A total of 197 children, or 55.6% of the eligible 3- to 7-year-old children from the larger cohort, completed the PRESS. Of the 44.4% ($n = 157$) who were not assessed, approximately half could not be located or contacted, and for about half the caregiver (i.e., foster parent, relative, or biological parent) refused to participate at the time self-reported depressive symptomatology was assessed. Finally, valid reports of depressive symptomatology could not be obtained from four children. Of the 197 children (93 boys and 104 girls) assessed, 89 (45%) were Anglo, 65 (33%) African-American, 38 (19%) Hispanic, and 5 (3%) were classified as other (e.g., Asian, Native American, Filipino).

Sample 2. The second sample included children who had been referred to a clinic for psychosocial treatment and who had participated in a pilot assessment program at this clinic (i.e., Chadwick Center, Children's Hospital and Health Center, San Diego). During the period from January, 1995 to January, 1996 an attempt was made to assess all children referred for treatment at the Center prior to their entry into treatment. More than half of the approximately 500 children who entered treatment were assessed. A total of 107 children between 3- and 7-years of age were administered the PRESS; 60.7% ($n = 65$) were females, with 58 (54.2%) identified as Anglo, 19 (17.8%) as African-American, 20 (18.7%) as Hispanic, and 10 (9.3%) as American Indian, Asian, or other. A total of 79 (73.8%) of the children had been referred for treatment because of sexual molestation. Maltreatment experiences of those 28 children who had not been molested included physical abuse ($n = 8$), neglect, or caretaker absence ($n = 10$), emotional abuse including witnessing domestic violence ($n = 15$), sexually aggressive behavior ($n = 4$), other inappropriate behavior ($n = 6$), and sibling of abuse victim ($n = 11$). Thus, these children had experienced multiple forms of maltreatment. (See Table 1).

Measures

For both samples, children between 3- and 7-years of age were administered the PRESS and their caregivers completed the Child Behavior Checklist (Achenbach, 1991). Additionally, a subsample of the Foster Care and all of the Clinic Referred children between the ages of 4- and 7-years were administered the Harter Pictorial Scale of Perceived Competence and Social Acceptance (Harter & Pike, 1984). Finally, the Peabody Picture Vocabulary Test-Revised (Dunn & Dunn, 1981) was completed by a subsample of the Foster Care sample.

Preschool Symptom Self-Report (PRESS). Martini et al. (1990) developed this pictorial scale to assess negative affect in young children. Two preliminary items are included to insure that children can respond to the demands of the scale. That is, the first item depicts an animal and a child, and the second a boy and a girl. A failure to point to the appropriate picture for either of these items (e.g., child asked to "point to the one that is more like you" after describing "this is a picture of a boy, and this is a picture of a girl") requires some brief instruction, and if still in-

TABLE 1. PRESS Means, Standard Deviations, and Percent Endorsing at Least One Negative Item by Socio-Demographic Factors for the Two Samples

		Foster Care			Clinic Referred	
	n	mean (sd)	%	n	mean (sd)	%
Total Population	197	3.41 (4.1)	68.5	107	3.89 (4.5)	77.6
Ethnic Group						
Anglo	89	3.88 (4.2)	76.4	58	3.71 (4.7)	79.3
Hispanic	38	2.95 (4.3)	65.8	20	2.95 (3.0)	75.0
African-American	65	2.97 (3.9)	60.0	19	4.89 (5.1)	78.9
Placement						
Biological Parent	22	3.27 (3.5)	68.2	-	-	
Relative	63	3.06 (4.0)	63.5	-	-	
Foster	112	3.63 (4.3)	71.4	-	-	
Gender						
Males	93	2.78 (4.0)	58.1	42	4.31 (4.7)	78.6
Females	104	3.97 (4.2)	77.9	65	3.62 (4.4)	76.9
Age						
3 yrs.	27	5.74 (4.9)	85.2	16	7.13 (5.1)	93.8
4 yrs.	40	5.10 (4.4)	82.5	23	4.74 (5.0)	82.6
5 yrs.	47	2.36 (3.7)	55.3	21	3.00 (4.1)	76.2
6 yrs.	40	2.95 (3.8)	72.5	25	2.88 (3.4)	84.0
7 yrs.	43	1.95 (2.8)	55.8	22	2.64 (3.7)	54.5

correct a second time, precludes presenting the scale to the child. The 25 items selected for the scale were based on an inspection of parental rating scales (e.g., CBCL) and symptoms for depressive disorders on the DSM-III-R.

Three additional items for the interviewer/observer were also developed. Specifically, following completion of the PRESS by the Foster Care sample, interviewers rated children (i.e., not at all, a little, most of the time) on three items indicating if they were sad/tearful, scared/withdrawn, and on task.

Pictorial Scale of Perceived Competence and Social Acceptance. Harter and Pike (1984) developed two 24-item versions of a pictorial self-perception scale. The versions, preschool-kindergarten and first-second grade, are typically administered to 4- and 5-year-olds, and 6- and 7-year-olds, respectively. Children respond to each item by first indicating which of two pictured individuals is "more like them" and subsequently describing the selected individual in the picture as being either "a lot like them" or "a little like them." Six different items, each scored on a 4-point scale, are combined to result in four subscale scores, two that assess perceived competence (e.g., cognitive and physical) and two that assess perceived acceptance (e.g., maternal and peer). Evidence of the reliability and validity of these two versions of this pictorial scale has been presented previously (e.g., Black, Dubowitz, & Harrington, 1994; Harter & Pike, 1984).

Child Behavior Checklist (CBCL). The parent version of the CBCL was developed as a rating instrument to assess social competence and behavioral problems in children and adolescents (see Achenbach, 1991 for a description of psychometric properties). Two forms were used in the present study. The first was designed for ages 2 and 3, and the second for ages 4- to 18-years. While there is considerable overlap between the 99 problem behavior items rated for the younger children and the 118 problem behavior items for the older children, there are some major differences (i.e., items included for the older children–e.g., sexual problems, sets fires, feels worthless or inferior; items excluded for older children–e.g., doesn't know how to have fun, gets too upset when separated from parents; and items worded differently–e.g., demands must be met immediately versus demands a lot of attention). Ratings for each of these two forms result in a number of normative scales (i.e., total behavior problems, broad-band internalizing and externalizing, and narrow-band). The younger version results in 6 narrow-band scores while the older version has 9 narrow-band scores. The CBCL has been used extensively in research studies with maltreated populations (e.g., Black et al., 1994; Mannarino et al., 1991).

Peabody Picture Vocabulary Test-Revised (PPVT-R). The PPVT-R is an individually administered measure of receptive vocabulary. Norms have been established and are utilized to obtain standardized scores including an IQ which is correlated with measures of intellectual functioning (Dunn & Dunn, 1981). Regardless, the PPVT-R should be considered a gross measure of verbal ability only.

Procedures

Foster Care Sample. As part of the larger short-term longitudinal study, children in the Foster Care sample and their caregivers were administered the PRESS and CBCL between 10- and 24-months (mean = 13.7) after the child had been removed from his or her home and had entered the Child Protective System. Assessments were scheduled with trained interviewers in the homes of the caregiver. A 2-month placement with the current caregiver was required so the CBCL could be completed. Informants were instructed to rate the frequency (never, sometimes, often) of each behavior from the CBCL over the past 2-months. At the time of these assessments (e.g., PRESS and CBCL), 22 of the 197 children had been reunited with their biological parent. The remaining 175 children were still in out-of-home placements, 63 with relatives and the remaining 112 with non-relative foster parents. A subsample of the 197 children ($n = 36$) was also administered the Harter Pictorial Scale of Perceived Competence and Social Acceptance. Finally, the PPVT-R was administered to 166 of the children at an additional assessment conducted approximately 5 months after removal.

Clinic Referred Sample. The Clinic Referred sample participated in a pilot assessment program that attempted to enroll clients (e.g., complete required forms, assign a medical record number), and assess children and their families prior to being assigned to a therapist. Trained psychology and social work graduate students interviewed children and caregivers individually. Children completed the PRESS and those who were 4 years of age or older also completed the Harter Pictorial Scale. Caregivers (over 95% were biological mothers) of the Clinic Referred children rated the frequency of behavior problems over the past 2 months on the CBCL.

RESULTS

Internal Consistency

Internal consistency on the PRESS for each of the two samples was found to be equivalent to that reported by Martini et al. (1990) (i.e., Cronbach's Alpha = 0.86 and 0.87). Breaking the larger Foster Care population into subgroups resulted in similar coefficients (0.86 to 0.89) across the three major ethnic groups (Anglo, Hispanic, and African-American), genders, and ages.

Concurrent Validity

Concurrent validity of the PRESS was assessed by determining its relationship to the Harter Pictorial Scale of Perceived Competence and Social Acceptance. For the smaller subsample of Foster Care children, none of the relationships reached significance, though correlations between PRESS scores and the subscales of Cognitive Competence and Peer Acceptance were $-.25$ and $-.33.$, respectively. When we examined the larger Clinic Referred sample, not only were these relationships found to be significant, but those between PRESS scores and the Physical Competence and Maternal Acceptance subscales were also significant. In all cases, greater perceived competence or acceptance was related to fewer self-reported depressive symptoms, consistent with findings reported for older children and adolescents (e.g., Smucker et al., 1986) (see Table 2).

Relationship of PRESS to Population Characteristics

Mean performance on the PPVT-R (85.6) revealed that the sample of Foster Care children scored almost one standard deviation below the norm. Scores ranged from 48 to 133 and the standard deviation (15.7) closely approximated the value used for standardization. The correlation between PRESS total scores and standardized scores on the PPVT-R for the sample of children who had been assessed on both measures was found to be negligible, $r(165) = -0.05$.

Summary descriptive statistics of responses to the PRESS for both samples are presented in Table 1. The overall sample means for the Foster Care and Clinic Referred samples were 3.41 ($sd = 4.1$) and 3.89 ($sd = 4.5$), respectively. As shown in Table 1, central tendency descriptors

TABLE 2. Concurrent Validity: Correlations Between Self-Reported PRESS Scores and the Harter Pictorial Scales of Perceived Competence and Acceptance for the Two Samples of Children

	Age Group		
	4-5 Year Old	6-7 Year Old	4-7 Year Old
Harter Cognitive Competence			
Foster Care Sample	−.33	−.28	−.25
Clinic Sample	−.33**	−.01	−.17*
Harter Physical Competence			
Foster Care Sample	0.13	−.03	0.03
Clinic Sample	−.30*	−.33*	−.32**
Harter Maternal Acceptance			
Foster Care Sample	0.10	−.21	0.11
Clinic Sample	−.38**	−.41**	−.33**
Hater Peer Acceptance			
Foster Care Sample	−.26	−.31	−.28
Clinic Sample	−.49**	−.61**	−.49**

Note. the sample sizes at each of the three age groups (4-5, 6-7, and 4-7) were 21,15, and 36, for the Foster Care sample, and 51, 34, and 85, for the Clinic sample, respectively.
*p < .05, **p < .01

were similar for the three major ethnic groups. Similarly, one-way analysis of variance indicated that the type of placement (i.e., biological parent, relative, or foster parent) was not related to PRESS responses in the Foster Care sample, $F(2,194) = 0.40, p = .67$.

PRESS total scores for each child in the Foster Care sample (range = 0 to 17) were subjected to a 2 (Sex: Male/Female) $\times$ 5 (Age: 3,4,5,6,7) analysis of variance. A significant main effect for Age emerged $[F(4,187) = 6.41, p < .01]$ with no significant main effect of sex and no significant interaction. Females in this population of young children tended to report more overall depressive symptoms than males (means = 3.97 and 2.78, respectively). A significant difference $[\chi^2 (1) = 8.94, p < .01]$ between females and males was found for the percent who endorsed at least one item on the PRESS (77.9% versus 58.1%). The tendency for females to score higher than males on overall PRESS scores can be accounted for by their being more likely to endorse at least one item since means for those females and males who endorsed at least one item were almost identical (5.07 and 4.84, respectively).

Examination of means presented in Table 1 and post-hoc comparisons indicate that the significant main effect for Age was due to the three older groups (5-, 6- and 7-year-old) reporting similar levels of depressive symptomatology that were significantly less than the younger two groups (3- and 4-year-old) who reported similar levels. Additionally, the percentage of children who endorsed at least one PRESS item was significantly related to age $[\chi^2 (4) = 14.9, p < .01]$. The two younger groups were more likely to endorse at least one item with the 5- and 7-year-old groups being least likely to endorse at least one item (see Table 1).

The age differences in overall PRESS scores cannot be attributed solely to differences in whether children did or did not endorse any items. That is, a similar 2 (Sex) $\times$ 5 (Age) ANOVA yielded a significant main effect for Age, $F(4,125) = 3.35, p < .05$, when only the 135 children who endorsed at least one item were included in the analysis. Post-hoc comparisons revealed the same pattern of responses, i.e., the 3- (mean = 6.74) and 4- (mean = 6.18) year-old groups had similar scores as did the 5- (mean = 4.27), 6- (mean = 4.07), and 7- (mean = 3.50) year- old groups, with the youngest group reporting significantly more depressive symptoms than the three older groups, and the 4-year-old group reporting more than the two oldest groups.

A similar 2 (Sex: Male/Female) $\times$ 5 (Age: 3,4,5,6,7) analysis of variance of the PRESS scores (range = 0-20) for the 107 children in the

Clinic Referred sample resulted in a trend for the main effect of Age only, $F(4,97) = 2.17$, $p = .078$. While not significant, the trend was consistent with what was found in the Foster Care sample. That is, the 3-year-old children tended to endorse the most items, with fewer items being endorsed among older children.

Relationship of PRESS to Maltreatment

Martini et al. (1990) reported that their group of Head Start students had a mean score of 5.75 on the PRESS. Children in the present Foster Care and Clinic Referred samples who were the same age (i.e., between 3- and 5-years-old) had comparable mean PRESS scores of 5.36 and 4.77, respectively.

For each of the Foster Care children assessed, information was obtained from case records indicating a single reason for the child's removal from his or her home. While it is possible that children experienced multiple forms of abuse and neglect, this single reason was recorded as the primary cause for the child protective system's involvement in removing the child. PRESS scores were subjected to a one-way analysis of covariance for three types of maltreatment (i.e., sexual abuse, physical abuse, and neglect/caretaker absent) with age and gender serving as the covariates. A significant main effect [$F(2,167) = 3.56$, $p < .05$] for type of maltreatment was found with adjusted PRESS means of 4.65 for the physical abuse group, 3.23 for the sexually abused group, and 3.03 for the neglect/caretaker absent group. Post-hoc multiple comparisons indicated that the source of this main effect was due to the physical abuse group reporting significantly more depressive symptomatology than the neglect/caretaker absent group. No other between-group comparisons were significant.

It was not possible to conduct the same analysis with the more homogeneous Clinic Referred sample (i.e., 73.8% sexually abused). A comparison of PRESS scores for those children who had been molested versus those who had experienced other forms of maltreatment resulted in a non-significant finding (means = 3.85 and 4.0, respectively).

Interinformant Agreement

In an effort to examine interinformant agreement about reported depressive symptomatology in these young children, relationships between PRESS scores (self-report), ratings made by the interviewers following observation of child responses on the PRESS (i.e., observer reports), and responses of the child's primary caregiver on the CBCL (i.e., caregiver reports) were examined.

Table 3 presents the correlations obtained between self-reported PRESS scores and caregiver reports on the CBCL for the three broad-band scales (Total, Externalizing, and Internalizing Problems) and for three narrow-band scales (Anxious/Depressed, Withdrawn, and Aggression). These three narrow-band scales were selected based on reviews identifying problem behaviors associated with childhood depression (cf. Kazdin, 1990). Additionally, the two versions of the CBCL were examined separately since we utilized raw scores as recommended by Achenbach (1991). Interinformant agreement between the 3-year-old groups from the two samples and their caregivers was in the low to moderate range, with only two correlations reaching significance (broad-band Externalizing Problems and total PRESS score [r (25) = 0.49, $p < .01$], and Aggression and total PRESS scores [$r(25) = 0.50, p < .01$] for the Foster Care sample). No evidence of agreement was found between the 4- to 7-year-old children in the two groups and their caregivers [$r's(167) = -0.03$ to $-0.09, p > .10; r's(90) = 0.06$ to $-.13, p > .10$, respectively].

For the Foster Care sample ($n = 192$), small but significant correlations were found between PRESS scores and observer ratings. Specifically, total PRESS scores were related to ratings of sad/tearful [$r(192) = 0.14, p < .05$] and on task/adequate attention [$r(192) = -0.12, p < .05$].

TABLE 3. Inter-Informant Agreement: Correlations Between Self-Reported PRESS Scores and Caregiver Reports on the CBCL for the Two Samples at Two Ages (3-Year-Old and 4- to 7-Year-Old)

	Foster Care PRESS Scores		Clinic PRESS Scores	
	3 Year Olds	4-7 Year Olds	3 Year Olds	4-7 Year Olds
Caregiver CBCL (*n*)	(25)	(167)	(10)	(90)
Total Behavior Problems	0.30	−.04	0.28	0.04
Internalizing Problems	0.26	−.09	0.33	−.11
Externalizing Problems	0.49**	−.05	0.14	0.06
Anxious/Depressed	0.28	−.09	0.30	−.13
Withdrawn	0.21	−.06	0.31	0.02
Aggression	0.50**	−.03	0.18	0.06

*p < .05; **p < .01

The negative correlation indicates that children who were rated as being less attentive reported higher levels of depressive symptomatology. While there was some indication that the 3-year-old group was responsible for these relationships, none of the correlations within this group reached significance [r'$s(25) = 0.23$ to $-0.31, p = .07$ to $.14$].

Finally, the relationship between reports from the two external observers (i.e., caregiver and interviewer/observer) was examined in the Foster Care sample. As with the prior analyses, these relationships were calculated for two groups of children (aged 3 and 4-7) since different versions of the CBCL were utilized and an unexpected pattern of relationships emerged previously (i.e., some evidence of inter-informant agreement was found for the 3-year-old children but not for the 4- to 7-year-old group). An examination of Table 4 shows that external informants (i.e., caregivers and interviewer/observers) were congruent in their ratings of affect for the 3-year-old group, i.e., sad/tearful ratings were significantly ($p < .05$) related to caregiver reports of Total Behavior, Internalizing and Externalizing Problems, as well as the three narrow-band Anxious/Depressed, Withdrawn, and Aggression Problems; and scared/withdrawn ratings were related to caregiver report of Anxious/Depressed problems. This was not the case with the 4- to 7-year-old group. None of the relationships reached the .05 significance level though some relationships approached significance, i.e., observer ratings of sad/tearful and caregiver reports of Anxious/Depressed [$r(164) = 0.13$, $p = .053$] and observer ratings of scared/withdrawn and caregiver reports of withdrawn behavior [$r(164) = 0.13, p = .052$].

The use of multiple significance tests for the correlations in Tables 2, 3, and 4 raises a question regarding the overall experiment-wise error rate. While multiple tests of significance legitimately raise this question, we would argue against this interpretation of our findings for the following two reasons. First, our results generally fit consistent, theoretically reasonable patterns that are independent of sample size. Second, many of the relationships we report lack sufficient power to support the argument that findings are largely due to inflated Type I error rates. For example, in Table 2, sample sizes for the foster care sample range from 15 to 36. The largest correlation in this group of comparisons is $-.28$, and is not reported as statistically significant. Based on a sample size of 36 the observed power to detect this value is only .37 ($\alpha = .05$, two-tailed). In contrast, the relationships for the clinic sample are based on sample sizes that range from 51 to 85. The smallest significant value in this group of relationships is $-.17$ and is based on a

TABLE 4. Correlations Between Caregiver Report and Observer/Interviewer Ratings by Age Group in the Foster Care Sample

	Ratings of 3 Year Olds ($n = 23$)			Ratings of 4-7 Year Olds ($n = 164$)		
	Sad	Scared	On Task	Sad	Scared	On Task
CBCL						
Total BP	0.43*	0.01	−.01	0.09	−.05	−.01
Int. Prob.	0.42*	0.33	−.09	0.10	0.09	0.01
Ext. Prob.	0.50**	−.08	0.15	0.11	−.10	0.02
Anx/Dep	0.39*	0.43*	−.09	0.13	0.11	0.04
Withdrawn	0.39*	0.19	−.08	0.06	0.13	−.06
Aggression	0.59**	0.06	0.22	0.11	−.11	0.02

*p < .05; **p < .01

sample size of 85. The power to detect this value is .34 ($\alpha = .05$, two-tailed). All of the remaining significant values are based on correlations of $-.32$ or stronger and are also reported as significant, regardless of sample size. Thus, rather than suggestive of a pattern of randomly significant findings produced by an inflated likelihood of Type I error or extremely high levels of power, our findings are both theoretically reasonable, and consistent with expectations based on rather modest power to detect significant relationships.

DISCUSSION

The results can be summarized as follows: (1) The Preschool Symptom Self-Report (PRESS) measure evidenced internal consistency in two groups of 3- to 7-year-old maltreated children, one who had been placed in out-of-home care and the other who had been referred to a mental health clinic. This consistency was maintained across gender, age, and ethnic groups. (2) Self-reported depressive symptomatology was related to self-reports of competence and acceptance by 4- to 7-year-old children in both a small subsample of the Foster Care children, and the larger sample of Clinic Referred children. (3) Responses on the PRESS were not related to an estimate of the children's verbal intelligence, type of current placement (e.g., biological parent, relative, or foster parent), or to ethnic differences. (4) Females in the Foster Care sample were more likely than males to endorse at least one item on the PRESS, but no differences in the number of items endorsed were evidenced across the two groups. (5) Younger children in the Clinic Referred sample tended to endorse more items, while in the Foster Care sample younger children were significantly more likely to endorse at least one item, and the 3- and 4-year-old groups endorsed more items overall than the 5-, 6-, and 7-year-old groups. (6) Overall means on the PRESS of children between 3- to 5-years of age in the two maltreated samples were equivalent to the mean reported by Martini et al. (1990) in a population of 3- to 5-year old Head Start students. This general observation is clarified by the finding that reports of depressive symptomatology in the Foster Care sample were related to the reason for their removal. Specifically, those children who were removed from their home for reasons of physical abuse reported more depressive symptomatology than those who were removed because of neglect or absence of their caretaker. And (7) Reports of affective disturbance by the child, caregiver, and an observer/interviewer tended to be concordant (child-caregiver, caregiver-observer/interviewer) for the group of 3-year-old children, but not for the 4- to 7-year old children.

The results of the current study along with Martini et al.'s (1990) report suggest that the PRESS is internally consistent across populations (i.e., Head Start/Maltreated, Gender, Ethnicity, and children 3- to 7-years of age). Contrary to claims that young children cannot understand items assessing cognitive symptoms, the present study found that young maltreated children responded to items in a consistent manner rather than randomly, as would be expected if they did not understand the items. Further support for the claim that responses of children to the PRESS are not influenced by verbal functioning (e.g., Martini et al., 1990) was obtained in the present study.

While evidence of the internal consistency of the PRESS and its independence from measures of verbal functioning had been previously presented by Martini et al. (1990), the present study provides the first evidence supporting the validity of this self-report measure. This evidence includes (1) the relationship found between reports of depressive symptomatology and perceived competence and acceptance, (2) the differential reports of depressive symptoms by children who had been removed from their home because of physical abuse, and (3) the relationship between self-reported depressive symptomatology and (a) caregiver-reported externalizing and aggressive problems and (4) interviewer/observer ratings of affect for the youngest children.

The significant relationships between measures attempting to assess depressive symptomatology and perceived competence/acceptance would be expected theoretically (e.g., Blatt & Humann, 1992; Kazdin, 1990) and are consistent with empirical findings with older children and adolescents (Kazdin, Moser, Colbus, & Bell, 1985). It is interesting to note that the peer acceptance subscale of the Harter appeared to have the most consistent relationship to reports of depressive symptomatology across the two samples. In contrast, there was a moderate relationship between reported depressive symptoms and maternal acceptance for the Clinic Referred sample, but no such relationship for the Foster Care sample was evident. It is not surprising to find this pattern given the fact that almost 90% of the Foster Care sample was living with a substitute caregiver while over 90% of the Clinic Referred children were living with their biological mothers.

A comparison group was not included in the present study. Nevertheless, an examination of self-reported depressive symptomatology of the Head Start children assessed by Martini et al. (1990) suggests that young maltreated children do not report more symptoms of depression than children not identified as maltreated. This suggested finding needs to be explored more fully in a study that includes appropriate comparison groups, a variety of measures including the PRESS, and outcomes that not only include a count of depressive symptoms but also identification of those children with a disorder.

The type of maltreatment that resulted in children entering the protective system was related to self-reported depressive symptomatology 1- to 2-years later. Specifically, children removed for physical abuse reported significantly more depressive symptoms than those who were removed because of neglect/caretaker absence. Thus, the PRESS was able to discriminate between children who were removed from their homes for different reasons. Additionally, the apparent inability of the PRESS to differentiate between the two maltreated samples and a Head Start sample could be attributed to the fact that some of the Head Start children may have experienced maltreatment, and/or combining children who experienced different types of maltreatment could mask differences between those exposed to specific types of maltreatment and those who were not maltreated.

It should be noted that child maltreatment researchers recognize how difficult it is to assess the type of maltreatment a child or adolescent was exposed to, much less to interpret what happened (Herrenkohl, 1990). In the present study we identified the type of suspected maltreatment that resulted in the child initially being removed from his or her home.

While this was not a direct measure of what the children experienced, we can assume that there was a high probability that this reported maltreatment reflected, in part, what happened to the children. A number of other studies (e.g., Allen & Tarnowski, 1989; Elliott & Tarnowski, 1990; Kaufman, 1991; Kazdin et al., 1985; Manly et al., 2001; Mannarino et al., 1991), utilizing other methods for determining type of maltreatment, report patterns of results that are consistent with the present findings. Thus, there is an accumulating literature, including the results of the present study, that suggests a history of physical abuse places children and adolescents at increased risk for self- and other-reported depressive symptomatology, relative to histories of neglect/caretaker absence, and non-maltreatment.

Efforts to establish the validity of the PRESS via examination of interinformant agreement met with mixed results. First of all, we found that ratings of an observer/interviewer following administration of the PRESS were significantly related to PRESS scores for the Foster Care sample, though the relationships were small. We found, as did Martini et al. (1990), that reports of primary caregivers in our Foster Care and Clinic Referred samples were not related to self-reports of depressive symptoms by children who were 4- to 7-years of age. On the other hand, we did find some support for interinformant agreement, and as a result, concurrent validity for the 3-year-old group. Specifically, caregiver-reported externalizing problems were related to self-reported symptoms on the PRESS for the Foster Care sample of 3-year-old children. Consistent with this pattern of self- and caregiver-reports were ratings by the observers/interviewers and reports by the primary caregivers that were related for the 3-year-old group but not for the group of 4- to 7-year-old children.

In a sample of 8- to 13-year-old children selected because they had a diagnosis of depression, Renouf and Kovacs (1994) found that interinformant agreement increased as the children got older. While at first glance this finding may appear to contradict the results of the current study, it is the case that the populations examined (e.g., diagnosed depression versus maltreated, 8- to 13-years-old versus 3- to 7-years- old), and measures used (selected items from the CDI and CBCL versus the total PRESS and established broad- and narrow-band scales from the CBCL) differed between the Renouf and Kovacs (1994) and the present study, respectively. Thus, it is possible that the findings of both studies are limited to the samples and measures that they utilized. On the other hand, an intriguing hypothesis emerges suggesting that there is a curvilinear relationship between age or developmental level and interinformant agreement about depressive symptomatology. Specifically, very young children may express their affect overtly through their non-verbal behavior, elementary school-aged children tend not to express affect non-verbally (or verbally), while preadolescents and adolescents may be more likely to begin sharing their affect with others.

In the present study gender effects were mixed. That is, no differences were found in the Clinic Referred sample, while girls in the Foster Care sample were more likely to endorse at least one item on the PRESS. Additionally, no differences in the number of items endorsed for the entire Foster Care sample, or for only those who endorsed at least one item were found. While this is the first report of gender effects on this measure for young children, it is consistent with reports for older children. Specifically, mixed results have been found when examining gender effects on the CDI (Kazdin et al., 1985; Saylor, Finch, Spirito, & Bennett, 1984) with girls tending to report more depressive symptomatology. In a study examining maltreated children, Kaufman (1991) found a trend for boys to be more likely to be categorized as depressed based on a structured diagnostic interview (Kiddie-SADS) than girls. Taking this apparent contradictory report and our findings into account, we might hypothesize that maltreated girls who do not have a mood disorder are more likely to endorse some items indicating depressive symptomatology than maltreated boys who do not have a disorder. As a result, more girls will report some depressive symptoms, and girls will tend to have higher scores on measures of depression that result in a count of depressive symptomatology. In contrast, on structured diagnostic interviews that result in individuals being identified as having a disorder, boys are at least as likely to be identified as depressed, if not more so, than girls.

Kaufman (1991) also reported that in her sample of 56 7- to 12-year-old children referred from Child Protective Services, children classified as depressed were older than the group classified as not depressed. Consistent age effects have not been reported for the CDI (Saylor et al., 1984). On the other hand, we did find that younger children were more likely to endorse an item indicating depressive symptomatology on the PRESS, as well as endorse more items than older children. These findings can be attributed not only to actual differences in depressive symptomatology, but also to characteristics of the younger children or the older children. For example, it is possible that the younger children could not respond to the cognitive demands of the measure (i.e., self-monitor and identify their feelings, decode descriptions of options presented verbally, and select an option that was most like them). If the younger children were unable to respond to the task demands of the measure, then we can assume that they responded randomly, with a position preference, or possibly to the pictures presented. This seems unlikely, however, because random or position responses would lead to (1) more items being endorsed than the overall mean of 15% found in the present study, and (2) lower levels of internal consistency than those found.

The inability of younger children to respond appropriately to the PRESS does not seem to be a plausible hypothesis since there was evidence that external reports of depressive symptoms in the youngest group were related to self-reported symptoms. In fact, external informants agreed with each other suggesting that the younger children may not only be reporting depressive symptoms accurately, but also expressing their affective or internal states overtly. That is, they may wear their emotions on their sleeves. Related to this explanation is the possibility that the older children were responsive to social demands (i.e., social desirability) and as a result were less likely to endorse items than the younger children who were not responding to such demands (i.e., they did not inhibit selection of clearly negative options on the measure). In any case, more information is required before we can make any definitive statements about the reasons for this observed age effect.

The focus of this descriptive study has been on the measure developed by Martini and his colleagues to assess depressive symptomatology in young children. While the present study is limited due to the lack of a comparison group, method for identifying maltreatment, and small sample sizes in some instances, evidence that the PRESS is a useful measure was obtained. Given the increased risk for developing internalizing problems in maltreated children and the potential to identify these problems early to target appropriate interventions, early assessment is critical. Martini and his colleagues recommend that a self-report measure should always be included when assessing affect in young children. Based on the results of the current study, we would suggest that the Preschool Symptom Self-Report (PRESS) may be particularly helpful when assessing young children who are suspected victims of maltreatment.

REFERENCES

Achenbach, T.M. (1991). *Manual for the Child Behavior Checklist and revised child behavior profile.* Burlington, VT: University of Vermont.

Allen, D.M., & Tarnowski, K.J. (1989). Depressive characteristics of physically abused children. *Journal of Abnormal Child Psychology, 17,* 1-11.

Barrett, M.L., Berney, T.P., Bhate, S., Famuyiwa, O.O., Fundudis, T., Kolvin, I., & Tyrer, S. (1991). Diagnosing childhood depression: Who should be interviewed– Parent or child? *British Journal of Psychiatry, 159,* 22-27.

Black, M., Dubowitz, H., & Harrington, D. (1994). Sexual abuse: Developmental differences in children's behavior and self-perception. *Child Abuse & Neglect, 18,* 85-95.

Blatt, S.J., & Homann, E. (1992). Parent-child interaction in the etiology of dependent and self-critical depression. *Clinical Psychology Review, 12,* 47-91.

Cohen, A.J., Adler, N., Kaplan, S.J., Pelcovitz, D., & Mandel, F.S. (2002). Interactional effects of marital status and physical abuse on adolescent psychopathology. *Child Abuse & Neglect, 26,* 277-288.

Digdon, N., & Gotlib, H.H. (1985). Developmental considerations in the study of childhood depression. *Developmental Review, 5,* 162-199.

Dunn, L.M., & Dunn, L.M. (1981). *Peabody Picture Vocabulary Test–Revised Manual.* Circle Pines, MN: American Guidance Service.

Elliott, D.J., & Tarnowski, K.J. (1990). Expressive characteristics of sexually abused children. *Child Psychiatry & Human Development, 21,* 37-48.

Harter, S., & Pike, R. (1984). The pictorial scale of perceived competence and social acceptance for young children. *Child Development, 55,* 1969-1982.

Herrenkohl, R.C. (1990). Research directions related to child abuse and neglect. In R.T. Ammerman & M. Hersen (Eds.), *Children at risk: An evaluation of factors contributing to child abuse and neglect* (pp. 85-108). New York: Plenum.

Hodges, K., Gordon, Y., & Lennon, M.P. (1990). Parent-child agreement on symptoms assessed via a clinical research interview for children: The Child Assessment Schedule (CAS). *Journal of Child Psychology & Psychiatry, 31,* 427-436.

Ialongo, N., Edelsohn, G., Werthamer-Larsson, L., Crockett, L., & Kellam, S. (1993). Are self-reported depressive symptoms in first-grade children developmentally transient phenomena? A further look. *Development & Psychopathology, 5,* 433-457.

Kashani, J.H., & Carlson, G.A. (1985). Major depressive disorder in a preschooler. *Journal of the American Academy of Child & Adolescent Psychiatry, 24,* 490-494.

Kaufman, J. (1991). Depressive disorders in maltreated children. *Journal of the American Academy of Child &Adolescent Psychiatry, 30,* 257-265.

Kazdin, A.E. (1990). Childhood depression. *Journal of Child Psychology & Psychiatry, 31,* 121-160.

Kazdin, A., Moser, J., Colbus, D., & Bell, R. (1985). Depressive symptoms among physically abused and psychiatrically disturbed children. *Journal of Abnormal Psychology, 94,* 298-307.

Kovacs, M., & Goldston, D. (1991). Cognitive and social cognitive development of depressed children and adolescents. *Journal of the American Academy of Child & Adolescent Psychiatry, 30,* 388-392.

Koverola, C., Pound, J., Heger, A., & Lytle, C. (1993). Relationship of child sexual abuse to depression. *Child Abuse & Neglect, 17,* 393-400.

Litrownik, A.J., & Steinfeld, B.I. (1982). Developing self-regulation in retarded children. In P. Karoly & J.J. Steffen (Eds.), *Advances in child behavioral analysis and therapy, Vol. 1* (pp. 239-296). Lexington: D.C. Heath.

Manly, J.T., Kim, J.E., Rogosch, F.A., & Cicchetti, D. (2001). Dimensions of child maltreatment and children's adjustment: Contributions of developmental timing and subtype. *Development and Psychopathology, 13*, 759-782.

Mannarino, A.P., Cohen, J.A., Smith, J.A., & Moore-Motily, S. (1991). Six- and twelve-month follow-up of sexually abused girls. *Journal of Interpersonal Violence, 6*, 494-511.

Martini, D.R., Strayhorn, J.M., & Puig-Antich, J. (1990). A symptom self-report measure for preschool children. *Journal of the American Academy of Child & Adolescent Psychiatry, 29*, 594-600.

Okun, A., Parker, J.G., & Levendosky, A.A. (1994). Distinct and interactive contributions of physical abuse, socioeconomic disadvantage, and negative life events to children's social, cognitive, and affective adjustment. *Development & Psychopathology, 6*, 77-98.

Renouf, A.G., & Kovacs, M. (1994). Concordance between mothers' reports and children's self-reports of depressive symptoms: A longitudinal study. *Journal of the American Academy of Child & Adolescent Psychiatry, 33*, 208-216.

Rosenfeld, A.A., Pilowsky, D.J., Fine, P., Thorpe, M., Fein, E., Simms. M.D., Halfon, N., Irwin, M., Alfaro, J., Saletsky, R., & Nickman, S. (1997). Foster care: An update. *Journal of the American Academy of Child & Adolescent Psychiatry, 36*, 448-457.

Rudolph, K.D., Hammen, C., & Burge, D. (1994). Interpersonal functioning and depressive symptoms in childhood: Addressing the issues of specificity and comorbidity. *Journal of Abnormal Child Psychology, 22*, 355-371.

Saylor, C.F., Finch, A.J., Spirito, A., & Bennett, B. (1984). The Children's Depression Inventory: A systematic evaluation of psychometric properties. *Journal of Consulting & Clinical Psychology, 52*, 955-967.

Silverman, A.B., Reinherz, H.Z., & Giaconia, R.M. (1996). The long-term sequelae of child and adolescent abuse: A longitudinal community study. *Child Abuse & Neglect, 20*, 709-723.

Smucker, M.R., Craighead, W.E., Craighead, L.W., & Green, B.J. (1986). Normative and reliability data for the Children's Depression Inventory. *Journal of Abnormal Child Psychology, 14*, 25-40.

Advances in the Reliability and Validity of the North Carolina Family Assessment Scale

Raymond S. Kirk
Mimi M. Kim
Diane P. Griffith

SUMMARY. *Objective*: Psychometric properties of the North Carolina Family Assessment Scale (NCFAS) are examined in relation to placement and prediction of future placement within the context of Intensive Family Preservation Services (IFPS). *Method*: IFPS workers recorded NCFAS intake and closure ratings for 1,279 families. The categorical rating data and change-scores are analyzed in relation to treatment outcomes and future placements. *Results*: Domain scores of the NCFAS remain highly reliable. Closure ratings are significantly related to placements and future placements of children, and change-scores are related to placements. *Conclusion*: The NCFAS is shown to be an instrument that helps practitioners assess areas needing service (i.e., parental capabilities, environment), documents

Raymond S. Kirk, PhD, Mimi M. Kim, PhD, MSW, and Diane P. Griffith, MA, are all affiliated with The University of North Carolina at Chapel Hill.

Address correspondence to: Raymond S. Kirk, PhD, School of Social Work, TTK Building CB# 3550, 301 Pittsboro Street, The University of North Carolina at Chapel Hill, Chapel Hill, NC 27599-3550 (E-mail: rskirk@email.unc.edu).

[Haworth co-indexing entry note]: "Advances in the Reliability and Validity of the North Carolina Family Assessment Scale." Kirk, Raymond S., Mimi M. Kim, and Diane P. Griffith. Co-published simultaneously in *Journal of Human Behavior in the Social Environment* (The Haworth Social Work Practice Press, an imprint of The Haworth Press, Inc.) Vol. 11, No. 3/4, 2005, pp. 157-176; and: *Approaches to Measuring Human Behavior in the Social Environment* (ed: William R. Nugent) The Haworth Social Work Practice Press, an imprint of The Haworth Press, Inc., 2005, pp. 157-176. Single or multiple copies of this article are available for a fee from The Haworth Document Delivery Service [1-800-HAWORTH, 9:00 a.m. - 5:00 p.m. (EST). E-mail address: docdelivery@haworthpress.com].

Available online at http://www.haworthpress.com/web/JHBSE
doi:10.1300/J137v11n03_08

changes, and relates the reported findings to placement and future place-ment. *[Article copies available for a fee from The Haworth Document Delivery Service: 1-800-HAWORTH. E-mail address: <docdelivery@haworthpress.com> Website: <http://www.HaworthPress.com> © 2005 by The Haworth Press, Inc. All rights reserved.]*

KEYWORDS. Family assessment, intensive family preservation ser-vices, placement, placement prevention, validity

This article presents new information on the reliability of the North Carolina Family Assessment Scale (NCFAS), the measurement of fam-ily functioning, and the concurrent and predictive validity (Rubio, Berg-Weger, Tebb, Lee, & Rauch, 2003) of the NCFAS in relation to placement prevention and future placement among families receiving Intensive Family Preservation Services (IFPS). The NCFAS shows growing promise as a practice-based instrument that assists practitio-ners in the identification of treatment needs of families referred for ser-vice, detecting and assessing treatment-related changes that occur in the NCFAS's measured domains, relating those changes to the placement status of children at the end of service, and in predicting the likelihood of the children's future out-of-home placement.

During the late 1970s the foster care population exceeded one-half million children. This growing population of children in out-of-home care led Congress to pass the Adoption Assistance and Child Welfare Act in 1980 (Public Law 96-272), which created a new national child welfare policy whereby child welfare agencies were required to "prevent unnec-essary placement and that in each case, a court must determine that the state has made reasonable efforts to prevent or eliminate the need for placement" (Ratterman, Dodson, & Hardin, 1987). A tacit requirement of this policy is that alternative services for families exist that render child removal "unnecessary." As a result of this requirement, a variety of ser-vices were expanded by child protection agencies to prevent out-of-home placement in the child welfare system, and new services were developed (Ratterman, 1986). These different types of family-based placement prevention programs include intensive home-based family treatment, family preservation services, home-based services, and fam-ily-centered child welfare services (Pecora & Fraser, 1992).

Beginning in the 1970s and concurrently with the implementation of Public Law 96-272 throughout the 1980s, IFPS was receiving widespread attention as a placement prevention program for high-risk families (Kinney, Haapala, & Booth, 1991). Pecora and Fraser (1992) describe IFPS as an intervention model based on Rogerian, cognitive-behavioral, crisis, and ecological theories, that views the family unit as the focus of service. Since its inception, IFPS has been associated with placement prevention. Research on the effectiveness of IFPS and other home-based service programs has usually focused on the number of placements prevented among children presumed to be at high risk of placement. However, this research has resulted in equivocal findings, and much of the research has been accompanied by discussions of poor targeting of high-risk families (Rossi, 1992; Shuerman, Rzipnicki, Littell, & Chak, 1993; Yuan, McDonald, Wheeler, Struckman-Johnson, & Rivest, 1990; USDHHS, 2001). The studies themselves are not without criticism. Numerous researchers have criticized the studies on the basis of design and methods (Pecora & Fraser, 1992; Fraser, Nelson, & Rivard, 1997; Heneghan, Horwitz, & Leventhal, 1996; Kirk, 2001) and on poor treatment model fidelity (Kirk, Reed-Ashcraft, & Pecora, 2002). However, targeting remains the most frequent criticism because the number of placements prevented is an inappropriate measure when families who receive the service are not at sufficiently high risk of placement. Furthermore, out-of-home placement may be the best case decision at the end of the brief intensive service period, and should not necessarily equate to service failure.

A term frequently used to describe sufficiently high risk to qualify for IFPS is "imminent risk" of placement. However, without knowing the factors that comprise imminent risk, use of the term may imply a false homogeneity of the intended treatment population. The literature reveals that there are numerous components of risk, or family dysfunction. Among the potential components of imminent risk are: weak family bonds, insufficient family skills and competencies, lack of formal and informal helping resources (Staudt, 1999); poverty (Eamon, 1994); substance abuse (Denby, 2001); and compromised mental health and/or mental capacity to participate in treatment (Berry, 1992). Bath and Haapala (1993) codified participating families according to type of maltreatment, as well as financial, medical, and personal stressors. This brief list suggests that various taxonomical approaches to describing treatment needs may be appropriate, as there are numerous ways to discuss family types, and numerous ways to measure family traits or characteristics when conducting research on IFPS or other family-based services.

Since the early 1990s many IFPS researchers have suggested that a more appropriate focus of research on these services should be improvements in family functioning (Pecora & Fraser, 1992; Pecora, Fraser, Nelson, McCroskey, & Meezan, 1995; McCroskey & Meezan, 1997; Reed-Ashcraft, Kirk, & Fraser, 2001; Denby, 2001; USDHHS, 2001). Pecora and Fraser (1992) have pointed out that the lack of standardized family functioning measures was, at the time, a significant limitation in IFPS research. Logically, changes in family functioning as a result of IFPS or other family-based services should relate to the end-of-service case decisions affecting placement regardless of the targeting of high-risk cases, a priori. However, prevention of placement remains a worthy policy objective, as long as family continuity can be maintained with deference to safety.

As Denby (2001) has suggested, program success should be measured according to improved family functioning and not merely placement avoidance, and research endeavors should focus on both treatment outcomes and treatment durability. Even the latest federal study of IFPS (USDHHS, 2001) concludes that future IFPS research should shift focus from placement prevention to improved child and family functioning, as well as identifying types of families most likely to benefit from the service. The NCFAS standardizes some relevant measures of family functioning, and is constructed in a way that supports IFPS and other family-based case practices, as well as assists in conducting research or program evaluation.

The following hypotheses will be tested in this study: (1) the NCFAS domains are sensitive to detecting change and will reflect the full range of ratings across the sample of families; (2) statistics relating to scale characteristics (reliability as reflected in Cronbach's Alpha, measures of central tendency, skewness and kurtosis) will be within acceptable ranges; (3) end-of-service (closure) scores will be significantly related to placement status, such that being rated at or above Baseline/Adequate at the end of service will be significantly related to non-placement, and positive change-scores will be significantly related to non-placement; and (4) intake ratings will be related weakly to placement status. This weak relationship is based on the logic that positive ratings at intake would not be expected to change during services, whereas negative ratings at intake would indicate a greater potential for change after services; and the pooling of variance among measures that would be expected to change with measures that would not be expected to change will mitigate the strength of potential predictive relationships.

METHOD

Design

This study employs a secondary analysis of a large sample to examine the relationships among the domain ratings on the NCFAS at intake and closure, and the concurrent and predictive validity of the domains with respect to out-of-home placement at the end of service and subsequent placement during the first year after referral for services. The validity of the Baseline/Adequate scale point as indicative of placement and future placement is explored, as are the full range of end-of-service ratings and change-scores.

The North Carolina Family Assessment Scale

The NCFAS is an instrument that provides ratings of family functioning on five domains: Environment; Parental Capabilities; Family Interactions; Family Safety; and Child Well-Being. The NCFAS was developed in the mid-1990s for use by IFPS practitioners to assess family functioning at the time of intake and again at case closure in order to assist caseworkers in the task of case planning, to measure treatment outcomes in the form of absolute ratings, and to calculate change–scores that provide an indication of progress that occurred or did not occur during the IFPS intervention. Each of the five domains and associated subscales utilizes a six-point rating scale that ranges from -3 (Serious Problem) to $+2$ (Clear Strength), through a "0" point labeled Baseline/Adequate. The Baseline/Adequate point is operationally defined as that point at or above which there is no legal, moral, or ethical reason to intervene, being determined by the combination of federal and state laws, judicial practices and community moral and ethical standards. Thus, the Baseline/Adequate rating may vary somewhat across jurisdictions and may evolve over time with changes in law and community standards.

The development of the NCFAS involved collaboration with a work group of IFPS providers, and was inspired, in part, by a common desire among practitioners, administrators and program evaluators to focus on various aspects of the IFPS intervention other than placement prevention. The NCFAS is a practice-based instrument designed to identify common themes of interest for practice with families in crisis. Subsequently, the Scale is categorized into measurement domains with scaling strategies that satisfy the requirements of the workers. The scales are capable of measuring family strengths as well as problems; to the extent possible, they avoid clinical jargon; they embrace clinical judgment of practitioners; and they are adaptable to parochial practice settings. The process of Scale development is described in greater detail in Kirk and Reed (2000).

The original validation study of the NCFAS was conducted in the late 1990s (Reed, 1998; Reed-Ashcraft et al., 2001). Reliability of the ratings was assessed using Cronbach's Alpha to test internal consistency (DeVellis, 1991), with alphas of .7 or higher being considered acceptable, and alphas of .8 or higher being considered to be strong. Construct validity of the domains was assessed by testing the relationship between domain scores on the NCFAS and scores from closely related constructs on other standardized instruments, including the Child Well-Being Scales (Magura & Moses, 1986), the Index of Family Relations (WAL-MYR, 1996), and the Family Inventory of Resources for Management (McCubbin, Thompson, & McCubbin, 1996).

Cronbach's Alphas for the intake ratings on retained items ranged from .76 to .93, and closure ratings ranged from .90 to .93. Correlations between NCFAS domain ratings and scores from comparison instruments were adequate for retained measures. The validation study is described in detail elsewhere (Reed-Ashcraft et al., 2001). The results of that study were used to finalize the present version of the NCFAS (Version 2.0), which is the subject of this continuing reliability and validity study.

Sample

Data were obtained from the statewide IFPS database, and include 1,279 families referred to IFPS by county departments of social services (DSS) served between July 1, 1999 and June 30, 2002. Because the NCFAS is required for all families served in the IFPS program, only eight families were eliminated from the analysis due to missing NCFAS data. Families referred to IFPS from sources other than DSS (e.g., mental health, juvenile justice) were not included because one-year follow-up data were not available. Data were collected by IFPS caseworkers from thirty-five programs serving fifty-four of North Carolina's 100 counties, and include family and service delivery information from the 4-6 week intervention period. Information includes: caretaker and child characteristics; basic demographics; risk of system placement; family strengths and problems; reasons for case closure; and placement information. Follow-up data for the

12-month period after referral to IFPS were available for 487 families whose service period ended by March 31, 2001, and whose children were matched in the statewide North Carolina Child Abuse and Neglect System (NCCANS).

Description of the Intervention

The IFPS intervention employed by the participating programs is based on the Homebuilder's Model. IFPS programs receive referrals for families with children who are at imminent risk of placement into systems of juvenile justice, social services, and mental health/developmental disabilities/substance abuse. The IFPS intervention model employs a short-term, crisis intervention with services provided primarily in the family's home or community. The intervention is available for a maximum of 6 weeks during which at least half of the caseworkers' time must be spent in face-to-face contact with the clients in their homes or communities. Policy guidelines for service include: improving family competence; building on family strengths and resources; providing services in a culturally competent manner; providing both therapeutic and concrete services; and sustaining small caseloads with a maximum of four families. Caseworkers are provided with specialized training to provide these specific services in accordance with the Homebuilder's training program.

Analyses

Using SPSS 11.5 to obtain all results, Cronbach's Alpha statistics are presented for each domain rating at intake and closure, illustrating the reliability of the domain ratings at both time periods. Statistics describing the domain distributions and properties of those distributions are presented and discussed. Descriptive statistics for the intake and closure ratings and change-scores on the five NCFAS domains are presented depicting the distribution of ratings across the sample of families at both time periods and the changes in those distributions associated with service. Change-scores were calculated for each domain, and the families in the sample were dichotomized on each domain at both intake and closure with the division point being a rating at or above Baseline/ Adequate versus any of the three problem categories. In practice the NCFAS scale ratings range from +2 (Clear Strength) to −3 (Serious Problem), but for analysis the data are converted to positive numbers ranging from 1 (Clear Strength) to 6 (Serious Problem). Categorical intake and closure ratings, the dichotomous categorical ratings, and the change-scores are cross-tabulated with placement at closure and placement within one year from the date of referral for service. The differences between expected and observed frequencies in the cross-tabulations are tested for statistical significance using the Pearson Chi-Square statistic.

RESULTS

Reliability of the NCFAS

The reliability analysis is based on the full sample of 1,279 families, and provides robust evidence that the NCFAS is reliable. Cronbach's Alpha for each domain at intake and at closure is presented below in Table 1. The Alphas at intake range from .72 to .90, and from .79 to .91 at closure. These results indicate that the subscales contribute substantially to the measured constructs and that the internal consistency is high (Nunnally, 1978). With respect to the original reliability and validity study of the NCFAS (Reed-Ashcraft et al., 2001), these results are confirmatory.

In addition to the internal consistency of the scales, the properties of the scale ratings are also important. The measures of central tendency and statistics relating to dispersion are presented in Table 2. The median

TABLE 1. Reliability of Scale Items for the Domains on the NCFAS (N = 1,279)

Domain	Time of rating	Number of scale items	Cronbach's alpha
Overall Environment	Intake	10	.90
	Closure	10	.91
Overall Parental Capabilities	Intake	7	.81
	Closure	7	.89
Overall Family Interactions	Intake	5	.79
	Closure	5	.81
Overall Family Safety	Intake	6	.72
	Closure	6	.79
Overall Child Well-Being	Intake	8	.78
	Closure	8	.81

TABLE 2. Measures of Central Tendency of Scale Ratings for the Domains on the NCFAS[1] (N = 1,279)

Domain	Time of rating	Mean	Median	Mode	Std. Dev.	Skewness[2]	Kurtosis[3]
Overall	Intake	3.52	3	3	1.48	.04	−.98
Environment	Closure	2.85	3	2	1.29	.53	−.37
Overall Parental	Intake	4.30	4	5	1.23	−.45	−.47
Capabilities	Closure	3.24	3	2	1.30	.39	−.62
Overall Family	Intake	3.99	4	4	1.34	−.18	−.76
Interactions	Closure	3.07	3	2	1.28	.40	−.51
Overall Family	Intake	3.98	4	4	1.36	−.25	−.64
Safety	Closure	2.92	3	3	1.28	.48	−.26
Overall Child	Intake	4.08	4	4	1.34	−.32	−.59
Well-Being	Closure	3.07	3	3	1.28	.41	−.44

[1]NCFAS categorical scores were converted for statistical analysis. They range from +1 (Clear Strength) to +6 (Serious Problem).
[2]The standard error for each skewness statistic = .07.
[3]The standard error for each kurtosis statistic = .14.

rating on each domain is either 3 or 4 in relation to a six-point scale, thus representing one of the two middle possibilities. Similarly, the means of ratings on all domains at intake and closure range from 2.85 to 4.3, with the standard deviations ranging from 1.23 to 1.48. These statistics suggest that the ratings are distributed across the full range of possible ratings, with means falling towards the problem ratings (values of 4, 5, and 6 in this analysis) at intake, but towards the baseline-to-strengths ratings at closure (values of 1, 2, and 3). These findings are consistent with the property of the scales to assist in the detection of changes in family functioning during brief interventions, and are confirmed by the skewness and kurtosis statistics. In each case, the skewness statistic is substantially less than 1.0, indicating that the ratings are sufficiently normally distributed across all domains at both intake and closure to provide measurement discrimination. Kurtosis values are also less than 1.0 and all are negatively signed, indicating that the distributions of ratings sufficiently retain the properties of a normal distribution but are slightly flattened. The slightly flattened distributions suggest that IFPS workers are taking advantage of the full range of rating options, not hesitating to utilize the end points of the scale, when appropriate.

Figure 1 provides a pictorial example of the distribution of ratings at intake and closure. The domain of Parental Capabilities is arbitrarily selected for this illustration. The light bars show the proportion of families at each rating at intake, and the dark bars show the proportion of families at each rating at closure. Although distributed across all possible ratings, the intake ratings reflect the slight negative skewness consistent with the fact that families in crisis tend to load on the problem-end of the scale. After service, the distribution of ratings still covers the full range, but also shows the slight positive skewness consistent with families having made progress during treatment.

Validity of the NCFAS

While a high degree of scale reliability has heuristic value, the true value of a reliable scale is only achieved after its validity is established. To determine the validity of the NCFAS in relation to the policy objective of placement prevention, the results of the domain ratings at intake and at closure were analyzed in relationship to the eventual case outcomes (placement at closure, placement within one year). There are

FIGURE 1. Percent of Families at Each Level of Functioning at Intake and Closure: Overall Parental Capabilities Domain (N = 1,279)

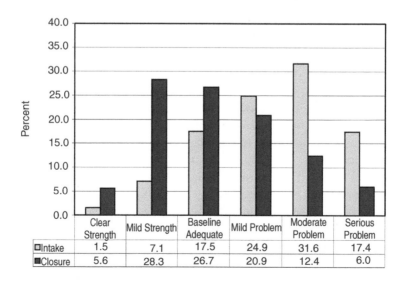

	Clear Strength	Mild Strength	Baseline Adequate	Mild Problem	Moderate Problem	Serious Problem
☐Intake	1.5	7.1	17.5	24.9	31.6	17.4
■Closure	5.6	28.3	26.7	20.9	12.4	6.0

several ways to conceptualize and analyze the data from the ratings. These different conceptualizations are presented in Tables 3 and 4.

Table 3 presents the descriptive statistics for the domain ratings. Both intake and closure statistics are presented, showing the percent of families rated across the full range of possible ratings. These are the categorical ratings assigned by workers, and the closure ratings may be conceptualized as the outcome measures, per se, for each domain of family functioning addressed by the NCFAS. For example, on the Environment domain, 8.9% of families were rated as having Clear Strengths at intake, and 13.7% are so rated at closure. This comparison indicates a modest increase in the number of families possessing clear strengths on this domain after service, compared to the number before service. The categorical ratings at intake can be cross-tabulated with placement to investigate predictive validity, and the categorical ratings at closure can be cross-tabulated with placement to investigate concurrent validity with placement at closure, and predictive validity for future placement (within 1 year from referral to IFPS).

A second alternative, also presented in Table 3, is to dichotomize families in relation to being rated at or above Baseline/Adequate or below Baseline/Adequate at intake or closure. For example, the table shows that a total of 51.1% of families were rated as being at or above Baseline/Adequate on the Environment domain at intake, and 72.4% were so rated at closure. This conceptualization is useful because the Baseline/Adequate rating is operationally defined as the point at or above which intervention should not be necessary. In theory, this dividing point should be related statistically to placement status at closure and to future placement. Indeed, as the NCFAS is a practice-based tool, the ratings are used to inform the placement decision and other case-closure decisions at the conclusion of IFPS services. However, cases are frequently closed without placement but with one or more domains remaining in the problem range of ratings. Thus, being rated below Baseline/Adequate is not a placement criterion, but rather is an indication of the possible need for ongoing services for problems that may or may not be observed at a level requiring child placement.

Finally, change-scores can be calculated by computing the difference between intake and closure ratings on the domains. However, the categorical nature of the NCFAS ratings requires that caution should be exercised with respect to attributing higher-order arithmetic properties to the data. In light of this caution, change is conceptualized in literal terms for subsequent analyses; either positive change, no change, or negative change may occur on each domain, thus retaining the categorical nature

TABLE 3. Descriptive Statistics for the Domains on the NCFAS[1] (N = 1,279)

Domain	Rating	Intake N	%	% at/ above or below baseline	Closure N	%	% at/ above or below baseline
Overall Environment	Clear S.	114	8.9		175	13.7	
	Mild S.	242	18.9	51.1	403	31.5	72.4
	Baseline A.	298	23.3		347	27.2	
	Mild P.	248	19.4		190	14.9	
	Moderate P.	240	18.8	48.9	122	9.5	27.6
	Serious P.	137	10.7		41	3.2	
Overall Parental Capabilities	Clear S.	19	1.5		72	5.6	
	Mild S.	91	7.1	26.1	362	28.3	60.7
	Baseline A.	223	17.5		341	26.7	
	Mild P.	318	24.9		267	20.9	
	Moderate P.	404	31.6	73.9	158	12.4	39.3
	Serious P.	222	17.4		77	6.0	
Overall Family Interactions	Clear S.	37	2.9		110	8.6	
	Mild S.	150	11.8	36.3	376	29.5	65.4
	Baseline A.	276	21.6		349	27.4	
	Mild P.	338	26.5		251	19.7	
	Moderate P.	278	21.8	63.7	139	10.9	34.6
	Serious P.	197	15.4		51	4.0	
Overall Family Safety	Clear S.	56	4.4		164	12.8	
	Mild S.	127	9.9	35.9	341	26.7	72.1
	Baseline A.	276	21.6		416	32.6	
	Mild P.	345	27.0		190	14.9	
	Moderate P.	279	21.8	64.1	116	9.1	27.9
	Serious P.	196	15.3		50	3.9	
Overall Child Well-Being	Clear S.	47	3.7		119	9.3	
	Mild S.	114	8.9	33.0	346	27.2	67.1
	Baseline A.	260	20.4		390	30.6	
	Mild P.	339	26.6		223	17.5	
	Moderate P.	307	24.1	67.0	141	11.1	32.9
	Serious P.	209	16.4		55	4.3	

[1]NCFAS categorical scores were converted for statistical analysis. They range from +1 (Clear Strength) to +6 (Serious Problem).

of the rating scheme. Table 4 presents these data. For example, the bottom row in Table 4 indicates that 39 families, or 3.1% of the sample, experienced a decline or negative change in Child Well-Being during the period of service, 33.9% did not experience change on this domain, and 63% experienced a positive change. It should be noted, however, that a positive change only indicates movement in the direction of improvement, and does not necessarily equate to being in the strengths range of ratings or being at or above the Baseline/Adequate rating at closure. For example, a positive change from Serious Problem to Moderate Problem would be a positive change of one scale increment, as would a change from Mild Strength to Clear Strength.

The results presented in Tables 5 through 7 demonstrate the concurrent and predictive validity of the NCFAS in relation to placement prevention. Table 5 presents the Pearson Chi-square significance tests resulting from the cross-tabulations using the NCFAS categorical ratings at intake and at closure with placement at the end of service (closure) and placement within one year of referral to IFPS services. Ratings in the strength ranges of the NCFAS at closure were significantly associated with non-placement at the end of service and at one year for each domain, while ratings in the problem ranges were significantly associated with placement. Again, this association is not surprising, as closure ratings are used to inform the placement decision, but do not determine the placement decision at the end of service. To a lesser degree, ratings in the strength ranges at intake were significantly related to non-placement at the end of service for all domains except Overall

TABLE 4. Change Statistics from Intake to Closure for the Domains on the NCFAS (N = 1,279)

Domain	Negative change		No change		Positive change	
	N	%	N	%	N	%
Overall Environment	51	4.0	613	48.0	614	48.0
Overall Parental Capabilities	33	2.6	350	27.4	893	70.0
Overall Family Interactions	49	3.8	436	34.2	789	61.9
Overall Family Safety	42	3.3	413	32.3	822	64.4
Overall Child Well-Being	39	3.1	432	33.9	802	63.0

TABLE 5. Contingency Table Results: NCFAS Categorical Ratings at Intake and Closure by Placement at Closure (N = 1,279), and Within One Year of Referral (N = 487)

Domain at intake	Placement status	Sig.	Chi-Square	df
Overall Environment	Placed at closure	p < .05	11.72	5
	Placed within 1year	p < .01	19.64	5
Overall Parental Capabilities	Placed at closure	p < .01	20.41	5
	Placed within 1 year	NS	--	--
Overall Family Interactions	Placed at closure	NS	--	--
	Placed within 1 year	NS	--	--
Overall Family Safety	Placed at closure	p < .05	11.65	5
	Placed within 1 year	NS	--	--
Overall Child Well-Being	Placed at closure	p < .05	12.58	5
	Placed within 1 year	NS	--	--
Domain at closure	Placement status	Sig.	Chi-Square	df
Overall Environment	Placed at closure	p < .001	77.40	5
	Placed within 1 year	p < .001	41.91	5
Overall Parental Capabilities	Placed at closure	p < .001	87.43	5
	Placed within 1 year	p < .01	16.84	5
Overall Family Interactions	Placed at closure	p < .001	78.42	5
	Placed within 1 year	p < .01	16.26	5
Overall Family Safety	Placed at closure	p < .001	105.50	5
	Placed within 1 year	p < .001	52.99	5
Overall Child Well-Being	Placed at closure	p < .001	97.14	5
	Placed within 1 year	p < .01	18.89	5

Note: NS = not significant

Family Interactions. With the exception of the ratings on the Environment domain, NCFAS ratings at intake were generally not predictive of placement outcomes within one year from referral. The term "prediction" is used here because the one-year placement data were actuarial data relating to the period following IFPS service closure, a period not influenced by ongoing casework by the IFPS program.

Table 6 presents similar findings using the dichotomous categorical ratings for the NCFAS domains. Intake ratings at or above Baseline/Adequate are not significantly associated with non-placement at closure, and only weakly associated with non-placement at one year for two do-

TABLE 6. Contingency Table Results: NCFAS Dichotomous Categorical Ratings[1] at Intake and Closure by Placement at Closure (N = 1,279), and Within One Year of Referral (N = 487)

Domain at intake	Placement status	Sig.	Chi-square	df
Overall Environment	Placed at closure	NS	--	--
	Placed within 1 year	p < .05	4.01	1
Overall Parental Capabilities	Placed at closure	NS	--	--
	Placed within 1 year	p < .05	4.61	1
Overall Family Interactions	Placed at closure	NS	--	--
	Placed within 1 year	NS	--	--
Overall Family Safety	Placed at closure	NS	--	--
	Placed within 1 year	NS	--	--
Overall Child Well-Being	Placed at closure	NS	--	--
	Placed within 1 year	NS	--	--
Domain at closure	**Placement status**	**Sig.**	**Chi-square**	**df**
Overall Environment	Placed at closure	p < .001	17.22	1
	Placed within 1 year	p < .01	8.83	1
Overall Parental Capabilities	Placed at closure	p < .001	27.79	1
	Placed within 1 year	NS	--	--
Overall Family Interactions	Placed at closure	p < .001	33.21	1
	Placed within 1 year	p < .05	4.92	1
Overall Family Safety	Placed at closure	p < .001	25.27	1
	Placed within 1 year	p < .001	17.98	1
Overall Child Well-Being	Placed at closure	p < .001	38.17	1
	Placed within 1 year	p < .01	6.76	1

Note: NS = not significant
[1]NCFAS dichotomous categorical ratings refer to the at/above or below Baseline/Adequate groupings displayed in Table 3.

mains, Overall Environment and Overall Parental Capabilities. In contrast, strong, significant associations were found with non-placement at the end of service and within one year for families rated at or above Baseline/Adequate at closure.

Table 7 presents the findings with respect to NCFAS change-scores. These results demonstrate strong, significant associations with non-placement at the end of service for families that experience positive change from intake to closure. Alternatively, families that experience

TABLE 7. Contingency Table Results: NCFAS Change Scores[1] from Intake to Closure by Placement at Closure (N = 1,279), and Within One Year of Referral (N = 487)

Domain	Placement status	Sig.	Chi-square	df
Overall Environment	Placed at closure	p < .001	20.86	2
	Placed within 1 year	NS	--	--
Overall Parental Capabilities	Placed at closure	p < .001	49.26	2
	Placed within 1 year	NS	--	--
Overall Family Interactions	Placed at closure	p < .001	45.09	2
	Placed within 1 year	NS	--	--
Overall Family Safety	Placed at closure	p < .001	52.61	2
	Placed within 1 year	p < .01	11.98	2
Overall Child Well-Being	Placed at closure	p < .001	45.30	2
	Placed within 1 year	NS	--	--

Note: NS = not significant.
[1]NCFAS change scores refer to the negative/none/positive groupings displayed in Table 4.

no change or negative change from intake to closure are significantly associated with placements at the end of service. However, changes in family functioning, either positive or negative, are not predictive of placement outcomes at one year for all domains except Overall Family Safety.

DISCUSSION

Results of this study support the efficacy of the NCFAS as a case practice tool to assist IFPS and other family-based workers to assess families for service planning, to reassess them at the end of service to document service outcomes and inform case closure decisions, and to obtain change-scores indicating progress resulting from service. The ratings obtained at the two measurement periods and the change-scores derived from them suggest that change is possible across all the measurement domains during the brief intervention periods typically associated with IFPS interventions.

Reliability statistics presented in Tables 1 and 2 confirm hypotheses 1 and 2. Ratings across all domains are normally distributed and kurtosis values indicate that the full range of ratings is routinely employed.

With one exception (Family Safety ratings at intake), alphas range from .79 to .91, which is a desirable range (DeVellis, 1991). Although still within the acceptable range, the alphas at intake and closure for Family Safety (.72 and .79, respectively) are considered by the authors to be high values because the full range of safety issues on the scale is not likely to apply to most families, depending on the type of child maltreatment associated with the family.

Hypotheses 3 and 4 are also confirmed, supporting the validity of the NCFAS in relation to placement status at the end of the IFPS intervention and within one year, although the strength of the relationships and the range of ratings that predict placement vary in informative ways. For example, the results from Table 5 indicate that the full range of ratings at closure is both significantly related to placement at closure and predictive of placement within one year. By contrast, the full range of intake ratings is only modestly related to placement at closure and generally not predictive of placement within one year.

These findings are important for two reasons that emerge when the results from Table 5 are compared to the results in Tables 6 and 7. First, the relatively weak capability of the intake ratings to predict placement at closure or thereafter, and the lack of predictive capability of the dichotomized intake ratings to predict placement at either time period (Table 6, upper half), suggests that the NCFAS should not be used as a device to screen out families from service at the time of intake. Rather, the closure ratings assigned using either the full range of ratings (Table 5, lower half) or dichotomized ratings (Table 6, lower half) suggest that even families with more serious problems at intake may experience enough positive change during IFPS to avoid placement at the end of IFPS service. Conversely, and in light of arguments made in the Introduction criticizing the use of placement prevention as an adequate measure of program success, even families having strengths on one or more domains at intake may not make enough progress in some other area or areas to avoid placement. In these cases the measured, documented absence of improvement may result in placement becoming the appropriate case decision and does not mean that IFPS failed to adequately serve the family.

Second, change scores in the positive direction (indicating improved family functioning), presented in Table 7, are associated with non-placement at closure, but positive change scores alone are not predictive of absence of future placement. However, for all domains except Overall Parental Capabilities, being at or above Baseline/Adequate does predict absence of future placement (Table 6). This finding suggests that whereas positive change alone seems to work in the short run, longer term family continuity may require evidence of greater change, or at least change equating to the Baseline/Adequate level of functioning. This knowledge should be helpful to social workers to identify families that may be able to remain together at the end of the time-limited IFPS intervention even with one or more domain ratings below Baseline/Adequate, but will need ongoing services in one or more areas to assure child safety and to continue the family's upward trajectory in terms of family functioning.

These findings also suggest that using a taxonomic approach, such as that used in the NCFAS, to identify strengths and problems in family functioning both supports case practice and addresses many of the concerns expressed by Berry (1992), Denby (2001), Pecora and Fraser (1992), Tracy (1991), Wells and Biegle (1992), the most recent federal study of IFPS (USDHHS, 2001) and others. A toxonomic approach can also help to identify the types of families most likely to benefit from IFPS and other forms of family-based services, and retain the benefits of service after the period of service.

Although the findings from the present study confirm the hypotheses under investigation and support previous reliability and validity studies of the NCFAS, additional research is needed. Preliminary analyses not presented in this study suggest that in addition to the occurrence of positive change, examination of the number of domains on which progress is made, the extent of progress made, and the particular combinations of problem areas at intake may also be predictors of placement and nonplacement. Further, although all of the statistical relationships involving placement that are discussed in this paper were in the expected direction, placement remains a relatively rare event both at closure and within one year. Thus, due to the increased number of variables under analysis in these questions and the assumptions underlying the requisite statistical analyses, much larger samples are required to explore these more complex and detailed relationships. More time is needed to amass samples sufficiently large to perform the analyses.

In conclusion, the results of the present study not only support the efficacy of the NCFAS as a case practice tool for social workers engaged in IFPS and other family-based services, they also inform us about the nature of the service population and the capacity of IFPS to address the treatment needs of those families. Employing a taxonomic approach to discussing and assessing family functioning may elucidate the presently amorphous concept of imminent risk, although we argue that focusing too narrowly on the relationship between imminent risk and placement prevention results in pedantic, academic arguments that divert attention from the practical matters associated with assessing and serving families in which child maltreatment has occurred.

REFERENCES

Bath, H.I., & Haapala, D.A. (1993). Intensive family preservation services with abused and neglected children: An examination of group differences. *Child Abuse & Neglect, 17*, 213-225.

Berry, M. (1992). An evaluation of family preservation services: Fitting agency services to family needs. *Social Work, 37*(4), 314-321.

Denby, R.W. (2001). Targeting the right families for family-centered services. In E. Walton, P. Sandau-Beckler, & M. Mannes (Eds.), *Balancing family-centered services and child well-being: Exploring issues in policy, practice, theory, and research.* New York: Columbia University Press.

DeVellis, R.F. (1991). *Scale development: Theory and applications.* Newbury Park, CA: Sage.

Eamon, M.K. (1994). Poverty and placement outcomes of intensive family preservation services. *Child & Adolescent Social Work Journal, 11*(5), 349-361.

Fraser, M.W., Nelson, K.E., & Rivard, J.C. (1997). Effectiveness of family preservation services. *Social Work Research, 21*(3), 138-153.

Heneghan, A.M, Horwitz, S.M., & Leventhal, J.M. (1996). Evaluating intensive family preservation services: A methodological review. *Pediatrics, 97*(4), 535-542.

Kinney, J., Haapala, D., & Booth, C. (1991). *Keeping families together. The Homebuilders Model.* New York: Walter de Gruyter.

Kirk, R.S. (2001). A critique of the evaluation of Family Preservation and Reunification Programs: Interim report. Retrieved May 2001, from http://www.nfpn.org

Kirk, R.S., & Reed, K.B. (2000). Designing and developing a new assessment and evaluation tool for family preservation service programs. In F. Jacobs, P. Hrusu Williams, J. Kapuscik, and E. Kates (Eds.), *Evaluating family preservation services: A guide for state administrators.* Medford, MA: Family Preservation Services Project, Tufts University.

Kirk, R.S., Reed-Ashcraft, K.B., & Pecora, P.J. (2002). Implementing family preservation services: A case of infidelity. *Family Preservation Journal, 6*(2), 59-82.

Magura, S., & Moses, B.S. (1986). *Outcome measures for child welfare services.* Washington, DC: Child Welfare League of America.

McCroskey, J., & Meezan, W. (1997). *Family preservation & family functioning.* Washington DC: CWLA Press.

McCubbin, H.I., Thompson, A.I., & McCubbin, M.A. (1996). *Family assessment: Resiliency, coping and adaptation. Inventories for research and practice.* St. Paul, MN: Family Social Science.

Nunnally, J.C. (1978). *Psychometric theory* (2nd ed.). New York: McGraw-Hill.

Pecora, P.J., & Fraser, M.W. (1992). Intensive home-based family preservation services: An update from the FIT project. *Child Welfare, 71*(2), 177-187.

Pecora, P.J., Fraser, M.W., Nelson, K.E., McCroskey, J., & Meezan, W. (1995). *Evaluating family-based services*. New York: Aldine de Gruyter.

Ratterman, D., Dodson, G., & Hardin, M. (1987). Reasonable efforts to prevent foster placement: A guide for implementation. American Bar Association, National Legal Resource Center for Child Advocacy and Protection. Washington, DC. *Children Today, Nov.-Dec.*, 26-32.

Reed, K.B. (1998). *The reliability and validity of the North Carolina Family Assessment Scale*. Chapel Hill, NC: The University of North Carolina at Chapel Hill.

Reed-Ashcraft, K.B., Kirk, R.S., & Fraser, M.W. (2001). The reliability and validity of the North Carolina Family Assessment Scale. *Research on Social Work Practice, 11*(4), 503-520.

Rossi, P.H. (1992). Assessing family preservation services. *Children & Youth Services Review, 14*(1,2), 77-97.

Rubio, D., Berg-Weger, M., Tebb, S.S., Lee, E.S., & Rauch, S. (2003). Objectifying content validity: Conducting a content validity study in social work research. *Social Work Research, 27*(2), 94-105.

Shuerman, J.R., Rzipnicki, T.L., Littell, J.R., & Chak, A. (1993). *Evaluation of the Illinois family first placement prevention program: Final report*. Chicago, IL: Illinois Department of Children and Family Services.

Staudt, M. (1999). Barriers and facilitators to use of services following intensive family preservation services. *Journal of Behavioral Health Services & Research, 26*(1), 39-53.

Tracy, E.M. (1991). Defining the target population for family preservation services. In K. Wells & D.E. Biegle (Eds.), *Family preservation services: Research and evaluation*. Newbury Park, CA: Sage Publications.

USDHHS (2001). *Evaluation of family preservation and reunification programs: Interim report*. Retrieved March 2001, from http://aspe.os.dhhs.gov/hsp/fampres94

WALMYR (1996). *The WALMYR assessment scale scoring manual*. Tempe, AZ: WALMYR.

Wells, K., & Biegle, D.E. (1992). Intensive family preservation services research: Current status and future agenda. *Social Work Research & Abstracts, 28*(1), 21-27.

Yuan, Y.Y., McDonald, W.R., Wheeler, C.E., Struckman-Johnson, D., & Rivest, M. (1990). *Evaluation of AB 1562 in-home care demonstration projects, volume 1: Final Report*. Sacramento, CA: Walter R. McDonald & Associates.

The Secondary Traumatic Stress Scale (STSS): Confirmatory Factor Analyses with a National Sample of Mental Health Social Workers

Laura Ting
Jodi M. Jacobson
Sara Sanders
Brian E. Bride
Donna Harrington

SUMMARY. The Secondary Traumatic Stress Scale (STSS; Bride, Robinson, Yegidis, & Figley, 2004) is an easy to administer 17-item

---

Laura Ting, PhD, is Assistant Professor, University of Maryland, Baltimore County, Department of Social Work.

Jodi M. Jacobson, PhD, is affiliated with Towson University, Family Studies Program.

Sara Sanders, PhD, is affiliated with University of Iowa, School of Social Work.

Brian E. Bride, PhD, is affiliated with University of Georgia, School of Social Work.

Donna Harrington, PhD, is affiliated with University of Maryland, Baltimore, School of Social Work.

Address correspondence to: Laura Ting, PhD, Assistant Professor, University of Maryland, Baltimore County, Department of Social Work, 1000 Hilltop Circle, Baltimore, MD 21250 (E-mail: LTing@umbc.edu).

[Haworth co-indexing entry note]: "The Secondary Traumatic Stress Scale (STSS): Confirmatory Factor Analyses with a National Sample of Mental Health Social Workers." Ting, Laura et al. Co-published simultaneously in *Journal of Human Behavior in the Social Environment* (The Haworth Social Work Practice Press, an imprint of The Haworth Press, Inc.) Vol. 11, No. 3/4, 2005, pp. 177-194; and: *Approaches to Measuring Human Behavior in the Social Environment* (ed: William R. Nugent) The Haworth Social Work Practice Press, an imprint of The Haworth Press, Inc., 2005, pp. 177-194. Single or multiple copies of this article are available for a fee from The Haworth Document Delivery Service [1-800-HAWORTH, 9:00 a.m. - 5:00 p.m. (EST). E-mail address: docdelivery@haworthpress.com].

Available online at http://www.haworthpress.com/web/JHBSE
doi:10.1300/J137v11n03_09

self-report measure of secondary trauma. Bride et al. (2004) reported a measure of three domains of traumatic stress specifically associated with secondary exposure to trauma: intrusion, avoidance, and arousal. The STSS was reported to have high levels of internal consistency reliability and indicated evidence of convergent, discriminant, and factorial validity. The purpose of this paper is to examine the reliability and validity of the STSS with a national, random sample of mental health social workers. To assess the fit of the data to the three-factor structure proposed by Bride et al., a confirmatory factor analysis was performed on data from 275 social workers who indicated exposure to client trauma. The model fit the data adequately although high factor intercorrelations strongly suggest a unidimensional scale. Subsequent confirmatory factor analysis of a unidimensional scale and a second order factor analysis yielded similar results. Findings indicate the need for further scale validation. Challenges remain for measuring and distinctly differentiating between secondary trauma symptoms of arousal, avoidance, and intrusion. Implications and suggestions for future research are discussed. *[Article copies available for a fee from The Haworth Document Delivery Service: 1-800-HAWORTH. E-mail address: <docdelivery@haworthpress.com> Website: <http://www.HaworthPress.com> © 2005 by The Haworth Press, Inc. All rights reserved.]*

KEYWORDS. Secondary traumatic stress, confirmatory factor analysis

Mental health professionals, specifically therapists working directly with clients and providing services to traumatized populations, are exposed to experiences and events through the lives of their clients. As many of these events are traumatic, the concern is that the therapists themselves may have increasing difficulty, both personally and professionally, in dealing with the accumulated trauma of such events. With this awareness in the field regarding the potential effects of secondary trauma, researchers and clinicians alike have become increasingly interested in researching this topic of secondary traumatic stress.

Research on the effects of secondary traumatic stress has been growing. Past research has shown that secondary traumatic stress, similar to vicarious trauma, compassion stress, or compassion fatigue (Figley, 1999, 2002; McCann & Pearlman, 1990), appears to be prevalent among mental health professionals. Specific estimates of trauma therapists experiencing post-traumatic symptoms are currently unknown; however, in the general population, the prevalence of post-traumatic stress disorder (PTSD) has been reported to be as high as 30% or more in observers and rescuers after serious accidents and disasters (Breslau, Davis, Andreski, & Peterson, 1991; Briere & Elliott, 2000; Bryant & Harvey, 1996; Duckworth, 1986; Figley, 1999, 2002). Gentry, Baranowsky, and Dunning (2002) note that all professional caregivers will at some point in their professional lives be forced to confront secondary traumatic stress and burnout. Working with traumatized clients indisputably has negative effects upon the mental health professional, including social workers.

Short term reactions to exposure to clients' traumatic materials include countertransference, while long term reactions include transformations of the professional's own cognitive schemas and beliefs, alteration of one's sense of trust and expectations of the world, as well as negative modifications of one's assumptions about others (McCann & Pearlman, 1990). Symptoms of vicarious traumatization include intrusive thoughts and images, avoidant behaviors and emotional numbing, withdrawal, fear, anger, anxiety, and depression. Vicarious traumatization changes are deemed to be permanent transformations within the therapist (McCann & Pearlman).

Figley (1999, 2002) notes that compassion fatigue is also a reaction from indirect exposure to a traumatic event. However, compassion fatigue develops as a result of the therapist's own empathy towards a traumatized client in addition to the therapist's own secondary experience of the traumatic material. While those suffering from PTSD and compassion fatigue often have identical symptoms and distress, the development of such empathetic reactions from the mere knowledge of or "learning of" the trauma without actual experience of harm or threat of harm is the hallmark of compassion fatigue (Figley, 2002).

Secondary traumatic stress also develops due to the secondary exposure to traumatic materials, but differs from compassion fatigue in terms of being the result of the stress from helping or wanting to help the traumatized client (Figley, 1999). Munroe (1999) has argued that due to the long term exposure to traumatic material through their work with clients, the resulting secondary reactions of compassion fatigue and stress within the helping professionals are similar to primary traumatic stress reactions from direct exposure. Intrusive thoughts or images, avoidant behaviors and emotional numbing, psychological distress and physiological somatic problems, hypervigilance, and arousal as well as impairment in daily functioning are all common negative reactions

(Brady, Guy, Poelstra, & Fletcher-Brokaw, 1999; Dutton & Rubenstein, 1995; Figley, 2002; Pearlman & MacIan, 1995).

The difficulty for researchers is to delineate between the conceptual differences of primary exposure to traumatic stress and secondary traumatic stress. Given that the signs and symptoms of secondary and primary traumatic stress are similar, the challenge remains in separating out which reactions are related to primary trauma exposure and which reactions are related to secondary trauma exposure.

MEASUREMENT OF SECONDARY TRAUMATIC STRESS

While the concept of secondary traumatic stress is familiar to researchers and clinicians, the ability to empirically measure such a phenomenon is still a challenge. Attempting to delineate between the symptoms of post-traumatic stress from direct exposure as opposed to indirect, secondary exposure to trauma is a formidable task. Researchers have developed scales to measure reactions to trauma; specifically, the original and revised Impact of Event Scale (IES; Horowitz, Wilner, & Alvarez, 1979 and IES-R; Weiss & Marmar, 1997) is designed to assess avoidant, intrusive, and hyperarousal symptoms post-trauma and has been widely used with trauma survivors (Horowitz, Wilner, & Alvarez, 1979; Weiss, 1996; Zilberg, Weiss, & Horowitz, 1982). The PTSD Symptom Scale (PSS; Foa, Riggs, Dancu, & Rothbaum, 1993) specifically measures and allows for the diagnosis of PTSD and is unlike the IES-R, which does not assess for the whole range of PTSD symptoms. The Traumatic Institute Stress Belief Scale (TSI; Pearlman, 1998) was developed to measure disrupted cognitive schemas due to traumatic experiences and vicarious traumatization. However, none of the instruments has been specific in its focus on measuring symptoms of secondary trauma.

Therefore, of specific interest to this study is a recent scale, the Secondary Traumatic Stress Scale (STSS; Bride et al., 2004), which was developed to measure the symptoms of secondary traumatic stress. The STSS measures the reactions of practitioners who have experienced traumatic stress through their work with clients by addressing the three factors of intrusion, avoidance, and arousal. However, Bride et al. provide the opportunity to measure secondary trauma specifically by defining "client exposure" as the traumatic event to which the mental health professional responds in the STSS.

The purpose of this study is to conduct psychometric analyses on the STSS (Bride et al., 2004), examining the internal consistency reliability as well as the factor structure through a confirmatory factor analysis (CFA) with a national sample of mental health social workers. Social workers, like their professional colleagues in other disciplines, have provided mental health services to traumatized populations and are at risk of developing secondary traumatic stress. The rationale for this study is based upon the fact that a brief, yet valid measure of secondary traumatic stress would be a valuable contribution to the field. The STSS would provide researchers with a necessary tool to measure such a complex construct and aid in the identification among mental health professionals of those who are at risk.

METHOD

Sample and Procedure

After receiving university IRB approval, data were collected from a national sample of mental health social workers. A random list of 1,000 social workers in the mental health subspecialty was generated from the National Association of Social Worker (NASW) database. This database contained approximately 50,000 self-designated mental health social workers throughout the United States. Self-designation of a mental health social worker and having a MSW degree were the two selection criteria for this study. The rationale was to focus on social workers who worked with the mentally distressed population and to exclude those who were not in direct practice with clients or who worked in settings that had minimal client contacts (e.g., teaching in higher education or in administration and research). Of the 1,000 mailed questionnaires, 515 were returned, comprising a 52% response rate. There were no follow-ups or reminders sent.

A five page self-report questionnaire was mailed to the sample. The cover letter defined the purpose of the study, assured complete respondent anonymity, and explained implied consent. A self-addressed, stamped return envelope was also provided.

The STSS was included in an anonymous self-administered survey as part of a protocol examining the reactions of mental health social workers who work with populations experiencing mental health issues and crises. Questions relating to perceived stress and secondary trauma reactions to client life events, including the impact of client suicide completions and attempts on the mental health of the social worker, were asked of the survey participants. Additionally, the survey included demographic questions and questions asking respondents about their methods of coping and the professional training they received.

Out of 515 surveys, the subsample used for this analysis was 275 respondents (53.3%) who completed the STSS, indicating they had experienced being impacted by their work with traumatized clients. Of the sample, over three-quarters (75.6%, $n = 208$) were female and 24.4% ($n = 67$) were male. The age of the respondents ranged from 25 to 70 years, with a mean age of 51 ($SD = 8.56$). The mean age of the sample is representative of the total NASW population (NASW, 2002). The majority of the sample was Caucasian (92%, $n = 252$). Over 90.5% ($n = 249$) had MSW degrees and 9.5% ($n = 26$) had PhD/DSW degrees. Almost half of the respondents were in private practice (46.2%, $n = 127$), and most worked with adult populations (86.9%, $n = 239$). The mean number of years of practice was 19 ($SD = 8.5$) with a range of experience from six months to 39 years. The clients who received services from these mental health social workers were predominantly female (59.3%, $n = 163$) with a mean age of 33, and had a diagnosis of affective/mood disorder (53.8%, $n = 148$).

The demographics reported are generally reflective of the total sample. T-tests and chi-square tests of significance were conducted to compare the STSS subsample and the non-STSS subsample. Results indicated that the mean age of the respondent, gender, race, and education level did not differ between the groups ($p > .05$). The only difference between the groups was the type of client population served. While both groups predominantly worked with adult clients, the subsample who completed the STSS served more adults than the non-STSS respondents (86.9% and 71.1% respectively, $p < .005$). See Table 1 for comparison of the samples.

Measure

Of specific focus in this study is the Secondary Traumatic Stress Scale (STSS; Bride et al., 2004). The STSS was developed using data from 287 social workers in a southeastern state in the United States. The STSS is a 17-item self-report measure administered in pencil and paper format (see Table 2 for items). Instructions for the STSS indicated that respondents should endorse how frequently an item was true for them in the past seven days. Responses ranged from 1 to 5 in Likert-form with 1 = never and 5 = very often. Of the 17 items, some are not stressor spe-

TABLE 1. Comparison of Sample Demographics

		CFA subsample	Non-respondents	t	x^2	p
		(n = 275)	(n = 240)			
Mean Age		51.73 (SD = 8.57)	49.94 (SD = 11.65)	−1.886		.06
Years Worked		19.05 (SD = 8.22)	18.52 (SD = 8.73)	−0.685		.49
Gender	Male	24.4% (n = 67)	22.4% (n = 50)		.258	.611
	Female	75.6% (n = 208)	77.6% (n = 173)			
Race	Caucasian	92.0% (n = 252)	87.9% (n = 197)		4.828	.437
	Other	8.0% (n = 22)	12.1% (n = 27)			
Highest Degree	MSW	90.5% (n = 249)	90.2% (n = 203)		.015	.903
	PhD	9.5% (n = 26)	9.8% (n = 22)			
Type of Clients	Adult	86.9% (n = 239)	71.1% (n = 160)		19.16	< .005
	Child	13.1% (n = 36)	28.9% (n = 65)			

Note. Due to missing data, not all numbers will equal to total *n*

TABLE 2. STSS Scale Items with Means, Standard Deviations (SD), and Subscale

Item	Subscale	Mean	SD
1. I felt emotionally numb	Avoidance	2.33	1.11
2. My heart started pounding when I thought about my work with clients	Intrusion	2.01	1.03
3. It seemed as if I was reliving the trauma(s) experience by my client(s)	Intrusion	1.81	.98
4. I had trouble sleeping	Arousal	2.04	1.01
5. I felt discouraged about the future	Avoidance	1.99	.98
6. Reminders of my work with clients upset me	Intrusion	1.93	.94
7. I had little interest in being around others	Avoidance	1.59	.82
8. I felt jumpy	Arousal	1.89	1.00
9. I was less active than usual	Avoidance	1.82	.96
10. I thought about my work with clients when I didn't intend to	Intrusion	2.60	1.04
11. I had trouble concentrating	Arousal	2.22	.99
12. I avoided people, places, or things that reminded me of my work with clients	Avoidance	1.67	.86
13. I had disturbing dreams about my work with clients	Intrusion	1.56	.81
14. I wanted to avoid working with some clients	Avoidance	2.10	1.09
15. I was easily annoyed	Arousal	2.08	1.01
16. I expected something bad to happen	Arousal	1.95	1.03
17. I noticed gaps in my memory about client sessions	Avoidance	1.71	.86

cific (items 1, 4, 5, 7, 8, 9, 11, 15, 16), but are general negative emotions and effects associated with traumatic stress (e.g., "I felt numb"; "I had trouble sleeping"). Other items (items: 2, 3, 6, 10, 12, 13, 14, 17) were specifically developed and worded using client exposure as the identified stressor (e.g., "My heart started pounding when I thought about my work with clients"; "Reminders of my work with clients upset me").

The STSS has three subscales: Intrusion (items: 2, 3, 6, 10, 13), Avoidance (items: 1, 5, 7, 9, 12, 14, 17), and Arousal (items: 4, 8, 11, 15, 16). Scoring is obtained by summing the endorsed frequency for each subscale as well as the total STSS scale. There is no reverse scoring.

Psychometric data for the original STSS indicated very good internal consistency reliability with coefficient alpha levels of .93 for the total STSS scale, .80 for the Intrusion subscale, .87 for the Avoidance subscale, and .83 for the Arousal subscale (Bride et al., 2004). Bride et al. demonstrated evidence for convergent and discriminant validity. Using structural equation modeling (SEM) techniques, Bride et al. performed a confirmatory factor analysis (CFA) to assess the question of factorial validity. Using select fit indices, and results from structural elements of the model such as factor loadings, t-values, squared multiple correlations, and factor intercorrelations, Bride et al. provided support for the three factor structure of the STSS.

Data Analyses

Cronbach's alpha was utilized to examine the internal consistency reliability of the STSS total scale as well as of the three subscales of Intrusion, Avoidance, and Arousal. In addition, a confirmatory factor analysis (CFA) was performed using LISREL 8.14 (Jöreskog & Sörbom, 1993) software to examine the fit of the data to the proposed three factor model.

A test of univariate normality indicated extreme kurtosis on several items of the STSS, thereby violating the normality assumption of structural equation models. Jöreskog and Sörbom (1993) specified the use of generally weighted least squares (WLS) as the estimation method with data that are non-normally distributed and ordinal in nature (as in the case of the Likert scale of the STSS). However, WLS requires a large sample size (> 400) that was not available in this study. Instead, this analysis utilized and compared both the maximum likelihood (ML) and generalized least squares (GLS) estimation methods with a covariance matrix. Without a large sample, ML and GLS were deemed the best methods to use under the circumstances (Hoyle & Panter, 1995;

Jöreskog & Sörbom, 1993). McDonald and Ho (2002), in comparing different estimation approaches, indicated that both ML and GLS methods seem to yield valid parameter estimates and associated statistics, despite non-normal data; therefore, ML and GLS methods seem to be "fairly robust against violations of normality" (p. 70).

Consistent with Bride et al.'s (2004) analysis, the following fit indices were used to assess the models' goodness-of-fit (see Table 4): the Goodness-of-Fit Index (GFI), the Comparative Fit Index (CFI), the Incremental Fit Index (IFI), and the Root Mean Square Error of Approximation (RMSEA). Additionally, as suggested by Byrne (2001) and Raykov, Tomer, and Nesselroade (1991), the Normed Fit Index (NFI), non-normed fit index (NNFI), and chi-square with its degree of freedom and p-value were also examined. In an ideal fit, the indices will all be greater than .90, RMSEA would be less than .080, and the chi-square would be non-significant with the ratio of chi-square to degrees of freedom less than two (McDonald & Ho, 2002).

Due to high factor correlations with the three-factor CFA, another CFA using a unidimensional model was tested and a subsequent second order factor analysis was also performed to assess the data. Fit indices are also reported in Table 4.

RESULTS

Internal Consistency Reliability

Internal consistency reliability for the total STSS 17-items was very high (α = .94) and was moderately high for the five-item Intrusion subscale (α = .79), the seven-item Avoidance subscale (α = .85), and five-item Arousal subscale (α = .87). Means and standard deviations are reported in Table 2.

Confirmatory Factor Analyses (CFA)

A confirmatory factor analysis (CFA) of the STSS (Bride et al., 2004) was performed (see Figure 1).[1] All items loaded significantly ($p <$ .05) on the factors identified by Bride et al. (2004); factor loadings ranged from .46 to .82 and t-values ranged from 9.27 to 15.12. All three factors were highly correlated with each other (Intrusion-Avoidance $r =$ .96, Intrusion-Arousal $r =$ .96, Avoidance-Arousal $r =$ 1.0).

FIGURE 1. Confirmatory Factor Analysis of the Secondary Traumatic Stress Scale with Three Factors

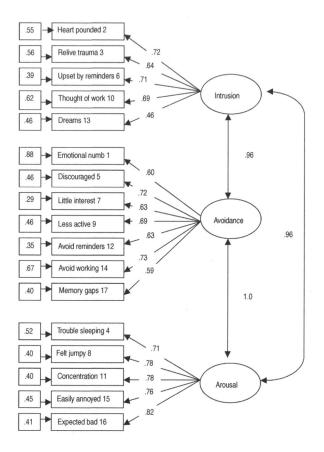

Note. The number in each indicator box is the item number on the STSS in TABLE 2.

The squared multiple correlations (R^2) for each observed variable represent the extent to which each individual item measures its underlying construct and to what extent the overall measurement model is represented by the observed measures (Byrne, 2001). For this model, the R^2 values ranged from .29 to .62 for the individual items, which indicated that between 29% and 62% of the variance on the items can be explained by its latent factor (see Table 3).

Multiple indices are reported as suggested by Byrne (2001) and Mc-Donald and Ho (2002) to examine different aspects of the overall model fit when parameters are tested simultaneously (see Table 4). While the Chi-square statistic is significant, indicating the observed covariation among the variables was not adequately accounted for by the model (Stevens, 2002), it is important to note that the Chi-square statistic is ex-

TABLE 3. Factor Loadings, T-Values, and Squared Multiple Correlations for the STSS Items in the Three-Factor CFA

Item	Intrusion	Avoidance	Arousal	t-value	R^2
2	0.72			12.58	0.49
3	0.64			11.52	0.43
6	0.71			13.91	0.57
10	0.69			11.59	0.43
13	0.46			9.59	0.32
1		0.60		9.27	0.29
5		0.72		13.44	0.53
7		0.63		14.29	0.57
9		0.69		13.23	0.51
12		0.63		13.54	0.53
14		0.73		11.93	0.44
17		0.59		12.33	0.46
4			0.71	12.82	0.49
8			0.78	14.79	0.60
11			0.78	14.78	0.60
15			0.76	14.06	0.56
16			0.82	15.12	0.46

TABLE 4. Fit Indices for Confirmatory Factor Analysis

Fit Index	Original model (Bride et al., 2004)	3-Factor CFA	One-factor CFA	Second Order CFA
χ^2	272.55	312.69	318.30	312.69
df	116	116	119	116
p	<.005	< .005	< .005	< .005
χ^2/df	2.35	2.69	2.67	2.69
GFI	0.90	0.88	0.88	0.88
NFI	N/A	0.88	0.88	0.88
NNFI	N/A	0.91	0.91	0.91
IFI	0.94	0.92	0.92	0.92
CFI	0.94	0.92	0.92	0.92
RMSEA	.069	.080	.079	.080

tremely sensitive to sample size, and with any large enough sample, a significant result will ensue. Therefore, other indices were taken into account. The GFI, which can range from zero to 1.0, with values closest to 1.0 indicating a good fit, at .88 is within the range of adequate. Values for the NFI, NNFI, CFI, and IFI were respectively .88, .91, .92, and .92, all indicating acceptable fit to the data. The RMSEA at .080 is considered a mediocre fit as values less than .080 indicate a good fit (Byrne, 2001; McDonald & Ho, 2002). After taking into account all the results, it appears that the findings provide support for the three factor structure of the STSS and the data fits the model adequately.

However, due to the high correlation results between the factors of Intrusion, Avoidance, and Arousal in the three-factor CFA, the possibility that secondary traumatic stress is a unidimensional construct was tested with another CFA (see Figure 2). There was no improvement of fit and fit indices were similar (see Table 4). A third CFA was conducted using Intrusion, Avoidance, and Arousal as first order factors and secondary traumatic stress as the second order factor (see Figure 3). Again, there were no differences on the fit indices (see Table 4).

DISCUSSION

With this sample, it is important to note that of the total respondents, over half (53.3%) acknowledged the effects of secondary trauma on their personal and professional lives. This is consistent with previous research findings on the prevalence of post-traumatic stress reactions among trauma therapists (Breslau, Davis, Andreski, & Peterson, 1991; Briere & Elliott, 2000; Duckworth, 1986; Figley, 1999, 2002).

While the data fit the three-factor model adequately, the high factor correlations between Intrusion, Avoidance, and Arousal suggest that there was difficulty in distinct differentiation between the constructs, although Bride et al. (2004) argued that given the theoretical nature of secondary traumatic stress, high correlations are to be expected. Current results are consistent with Bride's (2001) high factor intercorrelations using an analysis of covariance structures (Intrusion/Avoidance $r = .87$, Intrusion/Arousal $r = .94$, Avoidance/Arousal $r = .97$). However, when using a different method, by correlating the summated score totals of the respected subscales, slightly lower factor intercorrelations (Intrusion/ Avoidance $r = .74$, Intrusion/Arousal $r = .78$, Avoidance/ Arousal $r = .83$) were obtained by Bride et al. (2004). Due to these high intercorrelations, the possibility of secondary traumatic stress as a unidimensional

FIGURE 2. Confirmatory Factor Analysis of the STSS as an Unidimensional Scale

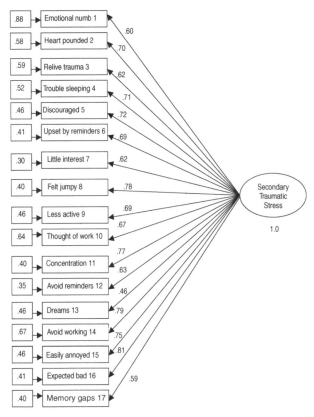

Note. The number in each indicator box is the item number on the STSS in Table 2.

construct was tested using a general, single-factor model. The results failed to show an improvement in the fit indices. The question of whether secondary traumatic stress has three distinct constructs or is one single construct remains to be further explored.

A third alternative interpretation is that the data are more adequately represented by a hierarchical factorial structure (Byrne, 2001), namely, the three first order factors of Intrusion, Avoidance, and Arousal are explained by a higher order factor, specifically secondary traumatic stress. Thus, the high covariation among the first order factors would be due to the regression on a second order factor. This possibility was tested with

FIGURE 3. Second Order Factor Analysis of the STSS with Intrusion, Avoidance, and Arousal as First Order Factors and Secondary Traumatic Stress as Second Order Factor

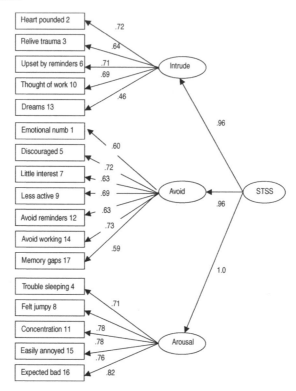

Note. The number in each indicator box is the item number on the STSS in Table 2.

another CFA. Again, the resulting fit indices were not different than those produced by the first order single-factor and three-factor models.

Conventional wisdom in the use of SEM suggests that the principle of parsimony be applied in model selection and fit assessment (Raykov & Marcoulides, 1999). For two models with comparable overall fit indices, the model with fewer free parameters is preferred (Mulaik, 1998). Thus, application of the principle of parsimony to the results of this study requires that the single-factor model of secondary traumatic stress be identified as the best-fitting model, suggesting that the STSS should be considered a unidimensional instrument. The internal consistency reliability for the overall STSS is high which also supports the idea of the scale as a unitary measure of secondary traumatic stress.

Strengths and Limitations

This study used a national random sample of sufficient size ($n = 275$) making the results more generalizable. The national sample is a strength and the first of its kind among social workers. However, as a result of the inclusion of only self-designated mental health social workers, there may be limitations in attempting to generalize the results to social workers in other areas of concentration, and to other types of mental health professionals in similar fields such as nursing, psychology, and psychiatry who provide services to traumatized clients.

The overall response rate of 52% is considered sufficient for survey research (Aday, 1996; Rubin & Babbie, 1997), but as with any type of research, there may be bias present (Anderson, Kasper, & Frankel, 1979). Specifically, of concern with this anxiety arousing topic is the issue of self-report bias. Those respondents with secondary trauma may be more or less likely to fill out the questionnaire, either because the topic may have been of personal importance to them or was a topic to avoid. Thus, non-response bias may have accounted for those who did not respond to the general survey or to the STSS.

Implications and Future Recommendations

While each of the three CFAs tested appeared to fit the model adequately, at this point, the high factor intercorrelations clearly favor a one-dimensional factor structure of the STSS. However, the adequacy of the fit for both the first-order and second-order, three-factor models, strongly indicates the need for future research to examine the conceptualization of traumatic stress symptomatology as multidimensional or unidimensional. Current findings of a unidimensional scale need to be validated. Future validation attempts with other samples are recommended to examine and determine the fit of data to the factor structure of the STSS originally proposed by Bride et al. (2004).

In addition to further investigation of the factor structure of the STSS, future research should examine the measure's ability to discriminate between secondary traumatic stress and other related constructs, specifically primary post-traumatic stress, as well as depression, which are commonly linked to avoidance and intrusion reactions. Another question of interest would be the predictive validity of the STSS on subsequent constructs of job dissatisfaction and burnout, as research indicates the high risk of developing such phenomena among mental health professionals suffering from traumatic stress (Figley, 1999, 2002).

This study represents an initial attempt to validate a new scale developed for the purpose of measuring secondary traumatic stress. The results did not provide strong support for Bride et al.'s (2004) conceptualization of the STSS as a three-factor structure. In fact, the factor correlation results raise questions about the STSS as a three-factor scale as originally hypothesized and strongly suggest a unidimensional scale instead. Despite these questions, the STSS is a short, easy-to-administer, self-report measure with promise and worthy of further validation and research efforts.

NOTE

1. While both the ML and GLS methods were used, the results were very similar; therefore, only the ML results will be reported to be consistent with the method used by Bride et al. (2004) in their original CFA.

REFERENCES

Aday, L. (1996). *Designing and conducting health surveys.* San Francisco: Jossey Bass.

Anderson, R., Kasper, J., & Frankel, M. (1979). *Total survey error: Applications to improve health surveys.* San Francisco: Jossey Bass.

Brady, J. L., Guy, J. D., Poelstra, P. L., & Fletcher-Brokaw, B. (1999). Vicarious traumatization, spirituality, and the treatment of sexual abuse survivors: A National survey of women psychotherapists. *Professional Psychology, Research, and Practice, 30,* 386-393.

Breslau, N., Davis, G. C., Andreski, P., & Peterson, E. (1991). Traumatic events and posttraumatic stress disorder in an urban population of young adults. *Archives of General Psychiatry, 48,* 218-222.

Bride, B. E. (2001). *Psychometric properties of the Secondary Traumatic Stress Scale.* Unpublished doctoral dissertation, University of Georgia, Athens.

Bride, B. E., Robinson, M. M., Yegidis, B., & Figley, C. R. (2004). Development and validation of the Secondary Traumatic Stress Scale. *Research on Social Work Practice, 14,* 27-35.

Briere, J., & Elliott, D. (2000). Prevalence, characteristics, and long-term sequelae of natural disaster exposure in the general population. *Journal of Traumatic Stress, 13,* 661-679.

Bryant, R. A., & Harvey, A. G. (1996). Posttraumatic stress reactions in volunteer firefighters. *Journal of Traumatic Stress, 9,* 51-62.

Byrne, B. M. (2001). *Structural equation modeling with AMOS: Basic concepts, applications, and programming*. Mahwah, NJ: Lawrence Erlbaum Associates.

Duckworth, D. (1986). Psychological problems arising from disaster work. *Stress Medicine, 2*, 315-323.

Dutton, M. A., & Rubenstein, F. L. (1995). Working with people with PTSD: Research implications. In C. R. Figley (Ed.), *Compassion fatigue: Coping with secondary traumatic stress disorder in those who treat the traumatized* (pp. 82-100). New York: Bruner/Mazel.

Figley, C. R. (1999). Compassion fatigue: Toward a new understanding of the cost of caring. In B. H. Stamm (Ed.), *Secondary traumatic stress: Self-care issues for clinicians, researchers and educators* (2nd ed., pp. 3-28). Lutherville, MD: Sidran Press.

Figley, C. R. (Ed.) (2002). *Treating compassion fatigue*. New York: Brunner-Routledge.

Foa, E. B., Riggs, D. S., Dancu, C. V., & Rothbaum, B. O. (1993). Reliability and validity of a brief instrument for assessing post-traumatic stress disorder. *Journal of Traumatic Stress, 6*, 459-473.

Gentry, J. E., Baranowsky, A. B., & Dunning, K. (2002). ARP: The accelerated recovery program (ARP) for compassion fatigue. In C.R. Figley (Ed.), *Treating compassion fatigue* (pp. 123-138). New York: Brunner-Routledge.

Horowitz, M., Wilner, N., & Alvarez, W. (1979). Impact of events scale: A measure of subjective stress. *Psychosomatic Medicine, 4*, 209-218.

Hoyle, R. H., & Panter, A. T. (1995). Writing about structural equation models. In R. H. Hoyle (Ed.), *Structural equation modeling: Concepts, issues, and applications* (pp. 158- 176). Thousand Oaks, CA: Sage.

Jöreskog, K. G., & Sörbom, D. (1993). *LISREL 8: Structural equation modeling with the SIMPLIS command language*. Chicago, IL: Scientific Software International, Inc.

McCann, I. L., & Pearlman, L. A. (1990). Vicarious traumatization: A framework for understanding the psychological effects of working with victims. *Journal of Traumatic Stress, 3*, 131-149.

McDonald, R. P., & Ho, M. R. (2002). Principles and practice in reporting structural equation analyses. *Psychological Methods, 7*, 64-82.

Mulaik, S. A. (1998). Parsimony and model evaluation. *Journal of Experimental Education, 66*, 266-269.

Munroe, J. F. (1999). Ethical issues associated with secondary trauma in therapists. In B. H. Stamm (Ed.), *Secondary traumatic stress: Self-care issues for clinicians, researchers, and educators* (pp. 211-229). Lutherville, MD: Sidran Press.

Pearlman, L. A., & MacIan, P. S. (1998). *The Traumatic Institute Stress (TSI) Belief Scale*. The Traumatic Stress Institute, South Windsor, CT.

Pearlman, L. A., & MacIan, P. S. (1995). Vicarious traumatization: An empirical study of the effects of trauma work on trauma therapists. *Professional Psychology, Research, and Practice, 26*, 558-565.

Raykov, T., & Marcoulides, G. A. (1999). On desirability of parsimony in structural equation model selection. *Structural Equation Modeling, 6*, 292-300.

Raykov, T., Tomer, A., & Nesselroade, J. R. (1991). Reporting structural equation modeling results in *Psychology and Aging*: Some proposed guidelines. *Psychology and Aging, 6*, 499-503.

Rubin, A., & Babbie, E. (1997). *Research methods for social work* (3rd ed.). Pacific Grove, CA: Brookes Cole Publishing Company.

Stevens, J. (2002). *Applied multivariate statistics for the social sciences* (4th ed.). Mahwah, NJ: Lawrence Erlbaum Associates.

Weiss, D. (1996). Psychometric review of the Impact of Events Scale-Revised. In B. H. Stamm (Ed.), *Measurement of stress, trauma and adaptation* (pp. 186-188). Lutherville, MD: Sidran Press.

Weiss, D., & Marmar, C. (1997). The Impact of Event Scale-Revised. In J. Wilson & T. Keane (Eds.), *Assessing psychological trauma and PTSD*. New York: Guilford.

Zilberg, N. J., Weiss, D. S., & Horowitz, M. J. (1982). Impact of event scale: A cross-validation study and some empirical evidence supporting a conceptual model of stress response syndromes. *Journal of Consulting & Clinical Psychology, 50*, 401-414.

Development of a Spiritual Support Scale for Use with Older Adults

Holly Nelson-Becker

SUMMARY. This study reports the development and empirical test of a measure of spiritual supports used by older adults in managing life challenge. The Spiritual Strategies Scale (SSS) consists of 18 items. Cronbach's coefficient alpha reliability for the measure was .86. The sample, gathered from interviews at four sites, consisted of 79 older adults who were predominantly Jewish European American and African American. Concurrent validity analyses suggest that this measure warrants further testing. This scale also has potential for clinical use in social work practice by counselors for older adults. *[Article copies available for a fee from The Haworth Document Delivery Service: 1-800-HAWORTH. E-mail address: <docdelivery@haworthpress.com> Website: <http://www.HaworthPress.com> © 2005 by The Haworth Press, Inc. All rights reserved.]*

KEYWORDS. Spirituality, religion, social work, scale, older adults, instrument

---

Holly Nelson-Becker, PhD, LCSW, is Assistant Professor, School of Social Welfare, The University of Kansas.

Address correspondence to: Holly Nelson-Becker, The School of Social Welfare, The University of Kansas, 1545 Lilac Lane, Lawrence, KS 66044 (E-mail: hnelson@ku.edu).

The author wishes to acknowledge the Council for Jewish Elderly (CJE), Chicago, IL for permission to interview residents in supported housing.

[Haworth co-indexing entry note]: "Development of a Spiritual Support Scale for Use with Older Adults." Nelson-Becker, Holly. Co-published simultaneously in *Journal of Human Behavior in the Social Environment* (The Haworth Social Work Practice Press, an imprint of The Haworth Press, Inc.) Vol. 11, No. 3/4, 2005, pp. 195-212; and: *Approaches to Measuring Human Behavior in the Social Environment* (ed: William R. Nugent) The Haworth Social Work Practice Press, an imprint of The Haworth Press, Inc., 2005, pp. 195-212. Single or multiple copies of this article are available for a fee from The Haworth Document Delivery Service [1-800-HAWORTH, 9:00 a.m. - 5:00 p.m. (EST). E-mail address: docdelivery@haworthpress.com].

Spiritual and religious resources are domains of support that may be especially meaningful to some of the current cohort of elders age 65 and above. A recent Gallup poll confirmed that 58% assessed religion as very important while 68% hold membership in a religious organization (PRCC, 2001). If older adults value religion both from an institutional and a personal perspective, then it is important for social workers to develop assessment tools for measuring the extent and the means by which religion and spirituality are engaged. In clinical intervention with older adults, religion and spirituality may not be mentioned unless the social work practitioner initiates the conversation. Some older adults, already feeling stigmatized by their use of therapy, believe that this is not a permissible part of their lives to discuss with a social work practitioner. An instrument customized to evaluate behavior encourages such conversations and offers a standard of measurement beyond the global question about the importance of religion and/or spirituality in the lives of older adults. Such a proposed measure is a first step in moving from measuring belief to identifying actions taken.

DEFINING RELIGION AND SPIRITUALITY

Religion and spirituality are broad terms that incorporate many meanings. Conversations have taken place across disciplines like psychology, theology, nursing, and social work to clarify what these terms comprise. Current interpretations are summarized below to provide a foundation for understanding the individual item construction in the SSS scale. This scale development study, part of a doctoral dissertation (Nelson-Becker, 1999), was directed toward building a functional definition of religion and spirituality.

Religion

Religion falls into three separate domains: the substantive, structural, and functional (Berger, 1974; Schabert, 1995). The substantive domain comprises the content of religious belief which has been a predominant research focus, but exploration into all aspects of religious domains is expanding (Batson, Schoenrade, & Ventis, 1993; Bergin & Jensen, 1990; Bullis, 1996; Canda & Furman, 1999; Joseph, 1988). Religious structures include physical objects (a statue of Buddha, a hymnal) or intangible social constructions (the ecumenical movement, the Sabbath) intricately related to sustaining both religious substance and function

(Schabert, 1994). The functional domain refers to both universal and personal purposes of religion. For example, religion may build a sense of community in a group or meet individual needs for socialization or guidance.

Religion has been interpreted to have affective and behavioral components and is assessed through a perceived relationship to whatever an individual declares the divine to be (James, 1902/1961). Rather than representing individual striving alone, religion encompasses fundamental consideration about the nature of being that may originate in an ultimate source (Tillich, 1963). Pargament (1997) agrees with this belief-based perspective of religion, but focuses on action, the human initiation of the quest, when he defines it as "a process, a search for significance in ways related to the sacred" (p. 34). His recent work has included measurement of religious coping (Pargament, 1999).

At one of the first White House Conferences on Aging, Moberg (1970) differentiated between the private and institutional spheres of religion that underscore structural and functional components. The private sphere included such behavior as prayer, meditation, and devotional reading while the institutional sphere was measured by church or synagogue attendance. Fundamentally, religion involves a community's formalized, institutional pattern of beliefs, practices, and values that focus on spiritual concerns (Canda & Furman, 1999; Nelson-Becker, 2003). Furthermore, a functional definition is concerned with how these ideas operate in the lives of individuals to meet needs and increase well-being.

Spirituality

Using the above typology for religion–substantive, structural, and functional–spirituality can also be conceptualized as having similar components, though perhaps fewer structural ones. However, spirituality may not be completely captured as a religious dimension. It is a human and transpersonal phenomenon expanding beyond traditional expressions of religious thought. Even Maslow (1970) designated a unique place for spiritual values in his slim volume, *Religion, Values, and Peak Experiences*. Spirituality has a universal nature that stands outside of more parochial definitions sometimes assigned by religion (Canda & Furman, 1999; Elkins, Hedstrom, Hughes, Leaf, & Saunders, 1988). The term spirituality has a Latin origin, "spiritus," or breath of life. Breath, a life-giving hallmark of humanity both functional and structural (symbolic), is consciously linked to spirit in some forms of meditative exercise. Just as breath is a sustaining part of physical being, so also is spirit. Structural components of spirituality beyond conscious breathing may include sacred objects such as a burning candle, or sacred spaces like a meditation garden, a beach at sunrise, an altar, or gathering with a faith community.

Spirituality is the "the human striving for a sense of meaning and purpose through moral relations between people and ultimate reality" (Siporin & Brower as cited in Canda, 1988, p. 39). Spirituality denotes a sense of journey, of becoming. Social work distinguishes between spirituality as essence and as one dimension among many (Carroll, 1998). Spirituality as essence refers to a core nature in humans that provides a sense of wholeness; spirituality as a dimension takes position next to biological, psychological, and social issues of the person.

Spirituality in aging is viewed as both the secular world of experience and the "sacred realm of the transcendent" (McFadden & Gerl, 1990, p. 35). For older adults, spirituality is an ongoing process of integration involving memory, experience, trust of others, anticipation, coping with a sense of mortality and connecting with a greater power. All of the changes experienced in the second half of life serve to sensitize elders to the need for self-reassessment and ultimately spiritual reintegration. This process of integration characterizes a functional approach.

MEASURING RELIGION AND SPIRITUALITY

Historically, from Leuba's 1916 and Thurstone and Chave's 1929 studies, measurement of spirituality focused on religious beliefs and expressions. Standard survey questions were asked about frequency of church/synagogue attendance and prayer, interpreted as degree of piety (Wulff, 1997). Currently, researchers from several disciplines focus their work on developing methods to operationalize these terms; to specify social and psychological correlates of religion; and to identify mediating factors (e.g., social support) that may provide competing explanations for diverse outcomes (Fetzer Institute, 1999; Hill & Hood, 1999).

Religiosity Measures

Thurstone developed a scale in 1929 to measure attitudes towards institutions of faith (Wulff, 1991; Wulff, 1997). This early measure successfully generated items that were differentially responsive to reported levels of church attitudes. Allport (1960) moved the work further by distinguishing between intrinsic and extrinsic religion in his Religious Orientation Scale. Intrinsic orientation was seen as a master motive that an individual sought to internalize and live fully. By contrast, an extrinsic orientation used religion for instrumental or utilitarian ends (i.e., security, fellowship). Critics of this scale noted that the orientations were complex, inadequately defined, and possibly confounded by personality. Yet this was a move forward in defining and measuring the functional value of religion (Wulff, 1997).

Batson and Ventis (1982) developed a Religious Life Inventory around three factors: religion as means, religion as end, and religion as quest. While two of the subscales augmented Allport's typology, the third attempted to measure open-endedness and concerns about ultimate life meaning. Other researchers suggested that this third "quest" factor failed to correlate with existing measures of religiousness, possibly measuring a stage along the lines of Fowler's stages of faith (Wulff, 1997). To further understand the dimensions underlying religious support, Ellison (1991) developed the Spiritual Well-Being scale that assessed components of religious and existential welfare. These measures recognize that religion as a construct may not answer all existential questions, but may be valuable for questions posed about ultimate life meaning.

Coping Measures

Spiritual support has been addressed conceptually through a more commonly used term of religious coping. Religious coping, too, has been a focus of instrument development. Koenig et al. (1995) used a Religious Coping Index (RCI) with a male sample of Veterans age 65 or older. He included an open-ended question about coping with stress, a rating of the extent that religion helped with coping, and an interviewer rating of respondent coping.

Pargament et al. (1988) identified three religious problem-solving styles: a self-directing style in which an individual takes responsibility for resolving the problem; a deferring style where the individual waits for solutions to emerge based on a Transcendent Power's/God's active efforts; and a collaborative style in which the individual works with God/Transcendent Force to resolve the problem. These types emerged from the 36-item Religious Problem-Solving Scale, delineating six phases of problem solving similar to D'Zurilla and Nezu's Social Problem Solving Inventory (1981): definition of the problem, generation of alternative solutions, selection of a solution, implementation, redefinition of the problem, and emotional self-maintenance. Neither the specific nature of the problems nor strategies used were addressed in this process-oriented study.

While religion includes the beliefs, rituals, and practices of a particular faith tradition, spirituality involves connections to a force beyond the self. Thus, spirituality may or may not include religious elements. Spiritual support may offer a richer and more pervasive frame for coping than a traditional, more institutional religious reference point. Measurement of spirituality in a way that considers how older adults pragmatically apply spirituality to solve problems offers promise in understanding how spirituality facilitates coping with the transitions of aging. Thus, development of a scale to measure behavior through spiritual support is timely.

METHOD

Item Selection and Development

The first step in the development of the Spiritual Strategies Scale was exploration of religion and spirituality related to the coping or problem solving process in older adults, detailed in the literature review. The second step involved generation of the item pool, indicators hypothesized to represent spiritual strategies older adults might engage. These strategies included affective, behavioral, and cognitive components.

Some items were broadly developed from themes in the scale items of Batson and Ventis (1982) and also Ellison (1991). Moberg's portrayal of private and public religious domains (strategies practiced alone or with others) led to a few items. Other items (later dropped due to confusion about the terms by this older adult sample) were built on Pargament's scale. Items such as leaving a legacy and assessing life were based on Koenig's (1994) conceptualization of spiritual needs of elders. A few items were generated out of the author's clinical experience with older adults. Redundancy of items was permitted initially in order to capture spiritual strategies in multiple ways. The items selected include a range of responses that individuals engage in their search for solutions to problems. Some items were conceptualized to capture most respondents (easy to endorse) while others would only capture a few individuals (hard to endorse).

Item Format

The item ratings were constructed on a five-point Likert-type scale with the following response anchors: Never, Rarely, Sometimes, Often, and Always. This five-point response set differentiates well among respondents and is relatively easy for respondents to recall. These response choices are both symmetrical and conceptually about equally spaced, though, of course, some subjectivity is involved in the choice. A stem using more modifiers may not lead to more accurate distinctions and greater sensitivity, particularly in an older adult sample.

The third step in the Spiritual Strategies Scale (SSS) construction was to field test the items with a group of 12 case managers who worked with senior adults. Some wording was changed, an item was refined into two separate components, and items with ambiguous or uncertain meanings were deleted. Two expert judges who were social work researchers/educators contributed to the final revision. They read the items for relevancy to the construct, clarity, and representative variety of dimensions.

Participant Sample

The fourth step in this scale development was to administer the items. Since the primary study question concerned exploring the ways older adults perceive and exercise spirituality and religion to manage life challenges, the sample sought was low income, ethnically diverse, and community dwelling. A relatively healthy sample was desired so responses about spiritual and religious domains would apply to adults aging normally, rather than individuals who might be viewed as seeking spiritual support in times of health crisis only. This investigation centered on four senior residential facilities, two situated on the north side and two on the south side of a large Midwestern city. The north side of this city is home to an affluent residential base that is becoming increasingly ethnically diverse, though less so in the two predominantly Jewish European American senior housing facilities selected. The two senior housing facilities located on the south side were less affluent and predominantly African American. All four sites were chosen because they met the sample criteria, and administrative permission for access was granted, though the initial goal to obtain lists of all residents in the four facilities was not attained.

The nonprobability available sample was determined by holding recruitment meetings at each site. A financial incentive of $5 was offered for completion of the interview. When the meetings initially failed to attract the desired numbers of participants, residents were approached in the apartment lobby and invited to participate. To capture the largest variety of respondents possible, the researcher varied recruitment times. Approximately 91% of older adults invited to participate eventually did agree to interviews. Appointments were scheduled and informed consent was obtained. The scale was given orally as part of a research interview for ease of administration in this older adult sample.

As interviewing progressed, the acceptance rate also increased, possibly due to a covert interviewee endorsement network. Men represented a smaller pool (38 of 122 tenants in one site) and had a somewhat higher refusal rate at all sites. It is likely that those who declined to participate may have been different from respondents.

Description of the Sample

The sample consisted of 79 respondents, 42 from the southern sites, and 37 from the northern sites. Median age was 78 with a range of 58 to 92 years. Median ages did not vary across the sites. The majority of respondents were female (n = 66, 84%) with equal percentages across the sites. Sixty-two percent had yearly incomes less than $10,000; another 29% reported income between $10,001 and $15,000. Median level of education across both groups was twelve years. Thirty percent attended church or synagogue weekly or more; 34% never attended. There was some sample variation in that southern site respondents were significantly more likely to attend a religious service [Chi-square (78) = 27.24; p < .000]. Ethnicity also represented a group difference: the northern sites were predominantly European American and Jewish while the southern sites were predominantly African American and Christian. Thirteen religious denominations were represented by this study. The highest percent was observant Jews (24.1%); self-identified cultural Jews (a mutually exclusive category) constituted 17.7%. Baptists comprised 16.4%, those who attended a community church were 7.6%, Catholics were 5%. Other denominations represented included African Methodist Episcopal (AME), Apostolic Church of God, and other Protestant denominations. One Buddhist who was African American participated. No affiliation was reported by 13.9%. The sample was small and represented two ethnically homogeneous groups. Thus, it is not representative of older adults generally.

DATA ANALYSIS

The data collected for this portion of a larger dissertation study was analyzed using SPSS. Highly intercorrelated items shown by the correlation matrix signal high individual item reliability (DeVellis, 1991). A corrected item total correlation correlates the item with all of the other scale items. Again, a high value is desirable. Large item variances are another important attribute that indicates that the item discriminates among respondents. Furthermore, an item mean that is near the center of the range of possible scores suggests that ceiling and floor effects are absent: the item is able to covary adequately with other items.

Cronbach's alpha coefficient was used for the reliability test. The alpha is a measure of the proportion of variance across scale scores that reflects the true score. A value of .70 is proposed by Nunnally (1978) as the lowest acceptable measure. A score between .80 and .90 is generally deemed very good. Longer scales require lower interitem correlations to achieve a high alpha. Thus, a shorter scale which is concisely written will measure the construct well and be less fatiguing for an older adult respondent. An exploratory factor analysis was conducted to determine properties of the SSS scale. One objective was to determine the percent of variation that could be explained. A second objective was to understand the meaning of the factors if groups of items appear to covary.

Pearson product-moment bivariate correlational analysis was used to assess convergent and construct validity. Convergent validity is a method of collecting evidence to support the validity of a scale by comparing results of the scale analysis with other measures that have established validity and reliability standards. While the validity of a construct can never be proven, it becomes stronger when correlated successfully with other instruments that function in different ways. The Life Satisfaction Index (LSI) developed by Neugarten, Havighurst, and Tobin (1961) was administered to this sample as well as the Geriatric Depression Scale (GDS) by Yesavage et al. (1983). While not representing exactly the same construct, it was hypothesized that some correlation would be evident, in a positive direction for the LSI and a negative direction for the GDS. Individuals who use a spiritual strategy for problem solving would do so repeatedly only because they perceive it as effective. If a spiritual strategy indeed does assist them in solving life difficulties, then there would likely be some correlation to life satisfaction or concurrent validity. Individuals who exhibit greater depression would be less motivated to apply spiritual strategies, thus those who score higher on depression should score lower on the Spiritual Strategies Scale (SSS).

The LSI measures psychological well-being and was designed for individuals over age 65. An estimate of split-half reliability at .79 was reported. A correlation of .79 was recorded with the Philadelphia Geriatric Center Morale Scale. The GDS has an alpha reliability of .94 and a one week test-retest correlation of .85 (Corcoran & Fischer, 1987). The GDS has shown concurrent validity of .83 with the Zung Self-Rating Depression scale and .84 with the Hamilton Rating Scale of Depression.

FINDINGS

Item Evaluation

The item analysis supports the logic of the SSS shown in Table 1. There were 18 items tested in the scale. The scale variances ranged from a low of 135 if an item was deleted to a high of 165. As discussed above, a high scale variance is desirable because it permits greater item discrimination. The corrected item-total correlation indicates an item's correlation to the rest of the scale excluding itself. If the item was correlated to the scale including all items, the correlation coefficient would tend to be inflated. The higher values express greater inter-item correlation. These indicate that the scale is more likely to reflect a variable common to each item. The items with lower values were assessing life, talking with friends about problems, accepting death, and providing service to others. These items may be measuring something other than spirituality. The column expressing the scale alpha reliability if an item is deleted confirms that the alpha would rise slightly if each of these four items were excluded.

Scale Reliability

When analyzed together the items achieved an alpha reliability of .8627 and a standardized item alpha of .849. The alpha measures internal consistency based on the average inter-item correlations of the scale. Alpha is influenced by both item covariation and length of the scale. An alpha of .8627 indicates that about 86% of the scale variance is systematic. This represents a good level of internal consistency. Since this scale contained 18 items, deleting the lower alphas did not greatly affect the total scale reliability. The individual item alphas varied from .842 to

TABLE 1. Item Analysis of the Spiritual Strategies Scale

N of Cases = 79; N of Items = 18, Alpha = .8627

Spiritual Strategy Items	Corrected Item-Total Correlation	Alpha if Item Deleted
1. Participate in religious community	.7687	.8401
2. Read spiritual literature	.7506	.8421
3. Participate in religious ritual	.6948	.8449
4. Pray	.6682	.8465
5. Look to God for life meaning	.6511	.8469
6. Practice a personal discipline	.5867	.8504
7. Look for meaning in night dreams	.5221	.8537
8. Watch religious t.v.	.5185	.8536
9. Meditate	.5086	.8542
10. Write in a journal	.4701	.8568
11. Forgive self	.4211	.8578
12. Leave a legacy	.3765	.8597
13. Forgive others	.3336	.8610
14. Participate in a support group	.3336	.8607
15. Provide service to others	.1949	.8649
16. Accept death	.1774	.8672
17. Talk with friends about problems	.1662	.8669
18. Assess life	.0920	.8677

.867. The scale was also analyzed using the 12 items with the highest inter-item correlations. This subset resulted in an alpha value of .8874.

Exploratory Factor Analysis

The scale was factor analyzed to evaluate whether subdimensions were present within the group of items. The Kaiser-Meyer-Olkin (KMO) measure of sampling adequacy tests whether partial correlations among variables are small. For this set of items, the correlation was .815. Values below .60 are not considered good prognostically for a scale, so this value supported the use of factor analysis. Bartlett's test of sphericity tests whether the correlation matrix is an identity matrix. Bartlett's test of sphericity gave a value of 555.505 at a significance level of p < .000. This indicated an adequate set of intercorrelations between items that supported factor analysis.

A principal components analysis (PCA) of the items resulted in six components with an eigenvalue over one (see Table 2). Together, they explained approximately 69% of the variance. A scree plot of the indicators verified that the first four explain the majority of the variance, 57.8%. The first component explained 32% of the variance, the second component 10% of the variance, and the third and fourth components each explained about 8% of variance. It is likely that some of the items were correlated with each other, since PCA extracts variance unique to the indicators as well as error variance.

Loadings of the item indicators on separate dimensions are presented in Table 3: a Religious component, a Social component, a Service component, and a Death Acceptance/Legacy component. An active/passive or public/private approach to measuring spiritual strategies did not separate into different dimensions as postulated. The 12 overtly religious items appeared to cluster together on the first component which is labeled Religious. The Social component (five items) consisted of assessing life, talking to friends about problems, joining a support group, and failing to forgive others or oneself. The Service component consisted of writing in a journal, providing service to others, and eschewing religious TV programs (three items). Accepting death and leaving a legacy constituted the fourth component (three items). A conservative criterion loading of .40 and above was applied. This is more stringent than a typical value of .30 and ensures a greater degree of confidence in factor loadings and variance, the square of the loadings.

Convergent Validity

Convergent validity with the Spiritual Strategies Scale was assessed together with the Life Satisfaction Index (LSI) using Pearson's r. This is

TABLE 2. Total Variance Explained

N = 79			
Component	Initial Eigenvalues	% of Variance	Cumulative %
1	5.800	32.222	32.222
2	1.827	10.151	42.373
3	1.407	7.815	50.189
4	1.376	7.643	57.832
5	1.075	5.975	63.807
6	1.028	5.710	69.516

TABLE 3. Spiritual Strategies Scale Component Loadings

N = 79

Item	Religious	Social	Service	Accept Death
Accept death				.710
Assess life		.617		
Forgive others		−.453		.407
Forgive self	.521	−.427		
Leave a legacy	.409			.530
Meaning dreams	.587			
Meaning/God	.744			
Meditate	.588			
Participate religious comm.	.841			
Participate religious ritual	.789			
Pray	.757			
Provide service to others			.539	
Read spiritual literature	.810			
Participate religious discipline	.689			
Support group		.501		
Talk w/friends re problems		.547		
Watch religious T.V.	.605		−.449	
Write in spiritual journal	.551		.432	

shown by Table 4. The Spiritual Strategies Scale (SSS) was significantly correlated with the LSI [R(78) = .556, p < .001], indicating that there was a moderate relationship. Concurrent validity was thus initially demonstrated with the LSI. This suggests that respondents who tended to employ spiritual strategies also experienced life satisfaction to a moderate extent.

Convergent validity was also measured by a negative correlation with the Geriatric Depression Scale (GDS) [r(78) = −.364, p < .01]. This result indicated that these older adults encountered somewhat less depression when they exercised spiritual problem solving approaches. The Religious subcomponent of the SSS mirrored results for the relationship of the complete scale to the LSI and the GDS. At least for the religious subcomponent, much of the correlation with the LSI was the same. The Social subcomponent had no relationship with either of the two measures, but both the Service and the Death Acceptance subcomponents had low to moderate positive correlations with the LSI and negative correlations with the GDS.

TABLE 4. Bivariate Correlations Among the SSS, the LSI, and the GDS

N = 79

Spiritual Strategies Scale (SSS) Components	Life Satisfaction Index (LSI)	Geriatric Depression Scale (GDS)
SSS complete scale	.556***	−.364**
Religious	.514***	−.257*
Social	-	-
Service	.345**	−.356**
Death Acceptance	.303**	−.411**

*p < .05; **p < .01; ***p < .001.

DISCUSSION AND APPLICATION TO SOCIAL WORK PRACTICE

Preliminary analysis of the Spiritual Strategies Scale indicated that the scale had a very good reliability with its high coefficient alpha of .86. This suggests some of the items were interrelated. It is no surprise that the highest intercorrelated items were those that were clearly religious in nature. These were items like participating in religious community and religious ritual, praying, and reading spiritual literature (which was often interpreted more narrowly by this sample as the Torah or the Bible). Individuals who were grounded in some form of religion had applied these approaches in their search for solutions to problems.

The term spirituality is less concrete than religion. Some of that ambiguity was present in the sample when they were asked in a qualitative question to describe what the word spirituality connoted for them and how they applied or expressed spirituality when they experienced problematic events or chronic difficulties. This suggests that spirituality and spiritual strategies are multidimensional to a greater extent than religion and religious problem-solving strategies. In fact, two other spiritual strategies not listed in this scale were proposed by respondents: renewing one's spirit in nature, and appreciating art and music. There are likely other items representing some form of spiritual action that could be included and tested in this scale when understandings of this dimension are enriched and deepened.

For this investigation, spirituality was conceptualized as a continuum from the more humanistic strategies to the overtly and unquestionably religious ones. However, the humanistic portion of the scale, talking to friends about problems and providing service to others, though they are symbolic of the connections that represent spirituality, do not clearly tap that component unless an individual interprets his/her own actions in this manner. Both of these items had low corrected item total correlations. Similarly, two items hypothesized to be particularly meaningful to an older adult, assessing one's life and accepting death, did not seem to be related to other spiritual and religious subcomponents. Older adulthood as a developmental stage offers some individuals an opportunity for spiritual reflection and synthesis; however, further work needs to be conducted to adequately tap these dimensions of aging in clinical assessment.

The factor analysis of the SSS indicated that four subcomponents had items that cluster in meaningful ways. The religious dimension included items that load at .40 and above. This subdimension comprised the greatest number of items in the scale (12) and most closely captured the concept. When reliability was assessed using only these items in the scale, the alpha reliability increased slightly.

Limitations and Future Research

The size of this sample was at a minimum level to test a new measure. In fact, it was somewhat lower than the size of 10 responses per ten items recommended by Stevens (1986). In a small sample, the covariation may not be stable or could be due to chance. Further, since this was an available sample and not a random one, it is subject to bias and does not represent a typical older adult population. This is true particularly because the sample was constricted by ethnicity and the faith affiliations identified by respondents. Initially tested with a predominantly Jewish European American and Christian African American sample, the SSS should also be used with other groups, perhaps with European and Hispanic Protestants and Catholics. Administration with a larger and more homogeneous sample would assist in validating these initial results. If it were administered to a group representing diverse world religions, other items should be developed and included.

A second issue is that this community dwelling sample evidenced relatively good mental health. Would a clinically depressed older adult sample such as might be found at a geriatric health or mental health center find spiritual problem solving strategies helpful? How might older adults with different health statuses employ these strategies? These questions are worthy of further consideration and testing.

In a self-report investigation there is always some question about congruence between cognition and behavior. Respondents may indicate they use a particular strategy, but this may not correspond to their actual behavior. They may not be fully aware of this dissonance between thought and action. Triangulation with other data sources such as family members could also confirm the assessment.

It is probable that the universality of this scale was limited because it was tested with primarily Judeo-Christian and nonaffili- ated respondents. Though one respondent was Buddhist and African American, her responses did not vary greatly from the mean on most items. Further items could be added to test a broader understanding by older adults of spiritual practices. Further work on this scale could include confirmatory factor analysis and Rasch analysis. Rasch is a logistic model of item response theory that involves the estimation of difficulty parameters and seeks to minimize item variance. It consists of a procedure to reveal whether a scale is internally consistent irrespective of trait variance in populations. Therefore, this method would be useful in a heterogeneous sample.

The test of convergent validity with the Life Satisfaction Index, while promising, is only one indicator of validity. Further tests of validity with other religious practice measures as they develop should be conducted.

CONCLUSIONS

Many older adults grew up in an era where a religious context was supported by family, community, and, in fact, the nation. Thus, religion/spirituality could be a more comfortable area for them to address than it is for a younger social worker who works with them. It is logical that older adults turn to religious and spiritual supports as one means of approaching the challenges in their lives. A scale such as this one enters new territory when it seeks to assess in a measurable way the behaviors that an older adult is already employing in the spiritual domain. In this study, unexpected amounts of qualitative data were gathered from discussion generated from the items. The Spiritual Strategies Scale thus has potential as a tool to elicit further discussion, for reinforcing current therapeutic practices, and for exploring new ones.

REFERENCES

Allport. G. (1960). *The individual and his religion: A psychological interpretation.* New York: Macmillan.

Batson, C., Schoenrade, P., & Ventis, W. (1993). *Religion and the individual.* New York: Oxford University Press.

Batson, C., & Ventis, W. (1982). *The religious experience: A social psychological perspective*. New York: Oxford University.

Berger, P. L. (1974). Some second thoughts on substantive versus functional definitions of religion. *Journal for the Scientific Study of Religion, 13*, 125-133.

Bergin, A. E., & Jensen, J. P. (1990). Religiosity of psychotherapists: A national survey. *Psychotherapy, 27*, 3-7.

Bullis, R. K. (1996). *Spirituality in social work practice*. Washington, DC: Taylor and Francis.

Canda, E. R. (1988). Conceptualizing spirituality for social work: Insights from diverse perspectives. *Social Thought*, Winter, 30-46.

Canda, E. R., & Furman, L. D. (1999). *Spiritual diversity in social work practice*. New York: The Free Press

Carroll, M. (1998). Social work's conceptualization of spirituality. *Social Thought, 18*(2), 1-13.

Corcoran, K., & Fischer, J. (1987). *Measures for clinical practice*. New York: The Free Press.

D'Zurilla, T. J., & Nezu, A. M. (1990). Development and preliminary evaluation of the social problem-solving inventory. *Psychological Assessment, 2*(2), 156-163.

Elkins, D. N., Hedstrom, L. J., Hughes, L. L., Leaf, J. A., & Saunders, C. (1988). Toward a humanistic-phenomenological spirituality: Definition, description, and measurement. *Journal of Humanistic Psychology, 28*(4), 5-18.

Ellison, C. G. (1991). Religious involvement and subjective well-being. *Journal of Health & Social Behavior, 32*, 80-99.

Fetzer Institute/NIA (1999). *Multidimensional measurement of religiousness/spirituality for use in health research*. Kalamazoo, MI: The Fetzer Institute.

Hill, P. C., & Hood, R. W. (1999). *Measures of Religiosity*. Birmingham, AL: Religious Education Press.

James, W. (1902/1961). *The varieties of religious experience: A study in human nature*. New York: Collier Books.

Joseph, V. (1988, Sept). Religion and social work practice. *Social Casework*, 443-452.

Koenig, H. G. (1994). *Aging and God: Spiritual pathways to mental health in midlife and later years*. New York: The Haworth Press, Inc.

Koenig, H. G., Cohen, H. J, Blazer, D. G., Kudler, H. S., Krishnan, K. R., & Silber, T. E. (1995). Religious coping and cognitive symptoms of depression in elderly medical patients. *Psychosomatics, 36*(4), 369-375.

Maslow, A. H. (1970). *Religion, values, and peak experiences*. New York: The Viking Press.

McFadden, S. H., & Gerl, R.R. (1990). Approaches to understanding spirituality in the second half of life. *Generations*, Fall, 35-38.

Moberg, D. O. (1970). Religion in the later years. In A.M. Hoffman (Ed.), *The daily needs and interests of the older person* (pp. 136-158). Springfield, IL: Charles C. Thomas.

Nelson-Becker, H. B (1999). Spiritual and religious problem solving in older adults: Mechanisms for managing life challenge. (Doctoral Dissertation, University of Chicago, 1999). *Dissertation Abstracts International*. (University Microfilms No. 9943099).

Nelson-Becker, H. B. (2003). Practical philosophies: Interpretations of religion and spirituality by African-American and Jewish elders. *Journal of Religious Gerontology, 14*(2/3), 85-99.

Neugarten, G. L., Havighurst, R. J., & Tobin, S. S. (1961). The Measurement of Life Satisfaction. *Journal of Gerontology, 16*, 134-143.

Nunnally, J. C. (1978). *Psychometric theory* (2nd ed.). New York: McGraw-Hill.

Pargament, K. I. (1997). *The psychology of religion and coping.* New York: Guilford Press.

Pargament, K. I. (1999). Religious/spiritual coping. In Fetzer Institute (Ed.), *Multidimensional measurement of religiousness/spirituality for use in health research* (pp. 43-56). Kalamazoo, MI: The Fetzer Institute

Pargament, K. I., Kennell, J., Hathaway, W., Grevengoed, N., Newman, J., & Jones, W. (1988). Religion and the problem-solving process: Three styles of coping. *Journal for the Scientific Study of Religion, 27*(1), 90-104.

Princeton Religious Research Center [PRRC] (2001). Importance of religion. *PRRC Emerging Trends.*

Schabert, V. F. (1995). Two models of religious commitment in coping and adjustment (Doctoral Dissertation, Stanford University, 1995). *Dissertation Abstracts International* (University Microfilms No. 9602954).

Stevens, J. (1996). *Applied multivariate statistics for the social sciences.* Mahwah, NJ: Lawrence Erlbaum.

Tillich, P. (1963). *Christianity and the encounter of world religions.* New York: Columbia University Press.

Wulff, D. M. (1991). *Psychology of religion: Classic and contemporary views.* New York: John Wiley and Sons.

Wulff, D. M. (1997). *Psychology of religion: Classic and contemporary views* (2nd Ed.). New York: John Wiley and Sons.

Yesavage, J. A., Brink, T. L., Rose, T. L., & Leirer, V. O. (1983). Development and validation of a geriatric depression screening scale: A preliminary report. *Journal of Psychiatric Research, 17*, 37-49.

Scale for the Identification
of Acquaintance Rape Attitudes:
Reliability and Factorial Invariance

G. Lawrence Farmer
Sarah McMahon

SUMMARY. Within the context of intimate interpersonal relationships, gender-based violence has a significant impact on the social-emotional functioning and development of women. Our ability to determine the effectiveness of our efforts to reduce sexual violence is linked to our ability to assess those attitudes that condone sexual violence. This study

---

G. Lawrence Farmer, MSW, PhD, is affiliated with the School of Social Work, Rutgers, The State University of New Jersey. Sarah McMahon, MSW, is Coordinator, Sexual Assault Services and Crime Victim Assistance, Rutgers, The State University of New Jersey.

Address correspondence to: G. Lawrence Farmer, Rutgers, The State University of New Jersey, School of Social Work, 536 George Street, New Brunswick, NJ 08904 (E-mail: glawrencefarmer@msn.com).

The preparation of this manuscript was supported by the Department of Sexual Assault Services and Crime Victim Assistance, Rutgers, The State University of New Jersey, and was partially funded by a grant from the New Jersey Department of Community Affairs, Division on Women, Office of the Prevention of Violence Against Women, Rape Care Program.

An earlier version of this paper was presented on January 20, 2001 at the Fifth Annual Conference of the Society for Social Work and Research.

[Haworth co-indexing entry note]: "Scale for the Identification of Acquaintance Rape Attitudes: Reliability and Factorial Invariance." Farmer, G. Lawrence, and Sarah McMahon. Co-published simultaneously in *Journal of Human Behavior in the Social Environment* (The Haworth Social Work Practice Press, an imprint of The Haworth Press, Inc.) Vol. 11, No. 3/4, 2005, pp. 213-235; and: *Approaches to Measuring Human Behavior in the Social Environment* (ed: William R. Nugent) The Haworth Social Work Practice Press, an imprint of The Haworth Press, Inc., 2005, pp. 213-235. Single or multiple copies of this article are available for a fee from The Haworth Document Delivery Service [1-800-HAWORTH, 9:00 a.m. - 5:00 p.m. (EST). E-mail address: docdelivery@haworthpress.com].

Available online at http://www.haworthpress.com/web/JHBSE
doi:10.1300/J137v11n03_11

examined the validity of college students' responses to the Scale for the Identification of Acquaintance Rape Attitudes (SIARA). The Scale for the Identification of Acquaintance Rape Attitudes is a measure designed to assess attitudes that are believed to be supportive of sexual violence within dating relationships. The sample consisted of 1,782 residential students in the first year class at a large, public university who participated in a sexual assault prevention program as part of a new student orientation. Exploratory and confirmatory factor analysis demonstrated that two dimensions, Sexual Expectations and Rape Mythology, could be used to characterize students' responses. Multi-group confirmatory factor analysis and mean structure analysis confirmed that the two dimensions provided equivalent measurements of the underlying construct for male and female subjects. Implications for the use of SIARA as a program outcome measure will be discussed. *[Article copies available for a fee from The Haworth Document Delivery Service: 1-800-HAWORTH. E-mail address: <docdelivery@haworthpress.com> Website: <http://www. HaworthPress.com> © 2005 by The Haworth Press, Inc. All rights reserved.]*

KEYWORDS. Sexual attitudes, college students, mean structure analysis, confirmatory factor analysis, acquaintance rape, date rape

Within the various contexts of social work practice, we find ourselves seeking to address the impact of exposure to interpersonal violence on the human development and social functioning of our clients (Danis, 2003; Humphreys & Thiara, 2003). The negative impact of rape and sexual assault on college students led to a 1992 amendment to the *Student's Right to Know and Campus Security Act of 1990.* This amendment, the *Campus Sexual Assault Victim's Bill of Rights*, requires institutions of higher education to make public data on sexual assaults and other crimes that occur on their campuses and to provide victim support services (Fisher, Cullen, & Turner, 2000). In response to legislation such as the *Campus Sexual Assault Victim's Bill of Rights*, many of the nation's colleges are combating interpersonal violence on their campuses with psycho-educational prevention and victim counseling programs (Black, Weisz, Coats, & Patterson, 2000; Hinck & Thomas, 1999). A common concern voiced about these programs is the lack of theoretically and methodologically sound measures of rape attitudes that can be used to assess the effects of these programs (Payne, Lonsway, & Fitzgerald, 1999). It is essential that as social workers become involved with the development and implementation of sexual assault prevention programs, we have the means to measure their impact on the sexual attitudes and beliefs of program participants.

This article will discuss findings from a factor analysis of the Scale for the Identification of Acquaintance Rape Attitudes (SIARA). This scale measures aspects of individuals' dating attitudes and beliefs that are believed to be associated with dating violence. The Scale for the Identification of Acquaintance Rape Attitudes was developed to address some of the problems identified in other measures of rape attitudes, particularly those in Burt's (1980) Rape Myth Acceptance Scale (Humphrey & Hillenbrand-Gunn, 1996). The Scale for the Identification of Acquaintance Rape Attitudes provides a measure primarily of young adults' attitudes towards rape, as it is likely to occur within the context of college dating relationships.

ACQUAINTANCE RAPE AND SOCIAL DEVELOPMENT

Acquaintance rape is defined as "nonconsensual sexual activity between persons who are engaged in a platonic, dating, marital, professional, academic or familial relationship" (Humphrey & Hillenbrand-Gunn, 1996, p. 5). Acquaintance rape is an international crime. A recent review of 50 international studies found that between 10 percent and 50 percent of women have experienced some act of physical violence by an intimate partner at some point in their lives (Venis & Horton, 2002). Much of that violence involves rape and/or sexual assault (Gender and Health Unit, 2003). Studies of college women provide evidence that a significant number of these women are finding themselves victimized in dating relationships (Fisher, Cullen, & Turner, 2000). The National College Women Victimization Study estimates that approximately five percent of college women are victimized in any given calendar year (Fisher, Cullen, & Turner, 2000).

Sexual assault and rape have a profound impact on the individuals' health and social-emotional functioning (Ambuel, Butler, Hamberger, Lawrence, & Guse, 2003; Rand & Saltzman, 2003; Tolan, Gorman-Smith, & Henry, 2003). Social learning and family theorists have linked exposure to gender-based violence to the future reproduction of violent interpersonal relationships (Hines & Saudino, 2002; Guttman, 2002), by the means of modeling and vicarious reinforcement represent processes within the family that promotes the reproduction of violent home environments (Hines & Saudino, 2002). Sexual assault, rape and other forms of domestic violence have been associated with heightened rates of depression, eating disorders, trauma symptoms, and self-harm among women (Ackard & Neumark-Sztainer, 2002; Humphreys & Thiara, 2003). A woman who is victimized by sexual violence is more likely to become a criminal perpetrator (Abel, 2001). Studies of female perpetrators arrested for domestic violence found that they were more likely to have histories of victimization than their male counterparts (Abel, 2001).

COMBATING ACQUAINTANCE RAPE

Anti-dating violence programs on college campuses use media campaigns, interactive psychoeducational workshops and psychodrama theater performances to change students' attitudes towards sexual assault (Holcomb, Savage, Seehafer, & Waalkes, 2002; Lonsway & Kothari, 2000; Schaeffer & Nelson, 1993). These programs are built on the premise that individual and collective attitudes regarding dating, courtship and sexual assault are important contributors to dating or acquaintance rape (Black, Weisz, Coats, & Patterson, 2000). A common concern voiced about these programs is the lack of theoretically and methodologically sound measures of rape attitudes that could be used to assess the effects of these programs (Payne, Lonsway, & Fitzgerald, 1999).

Presently the Scale for the Identification of Acquaintance Rape Attitudes (SIARA) is the only measure of rape attitudes targeting acquaintance rapes that occur within the context of college dating relationships (Humphrey & Hillenbrand-Gunn, 1996). To date, there has been only one study conducted assessing the psychometric properties of the SIARA (Humphrey & Hillenbrand-Gunn, 1996). Humphrey and Hillenbrand-Gunn (1996) conducted an exploratory factor analysis of the scale using a sample of 338 college participants drawn from introductory psychology classes at a mid-western university. The authors concluded that the scale was best represented by a one-factor structure containing thirty-three items. Whether this measure effectively assesses the impact of anti-rape prevention programs will be known only through further research. It is particularly important that validity studies of the measure examine potential gender differences. Previous research on the sexual scripts that guide interpersonal conduct between men and women highlights the importance of developing measures that are sensitive to gender differences (Muehlenhard & Rodgers, 1998). For example, studies of "token resistance," i.e., refusing or resisting sexual activity while intending to engage in that activity, indicate differences in opinion between men and women regarding how often women engage in this type of behavior (Muehlenhard & Rodgers, 1998).

This study seeks to replicate and extend Humphrey and Hillenbrand-Gunn's (1996) initial findings by addressing the following questions: Can the findings of the Humphrey and Hillenbrand-Gunn (1996) study indicating the unidimensionality of the SIARA be replicated? Are there differences in the factor structure of the SIARA between male and female college students?

METHODOLOGY

Sampling

The sample size before listwise deletion was 2,163 which represented a response rate of ninety-one percent. After listwise deletion, the study sample consisted of 1,782 residential students in the first-year class at a large, public university who were required to participate in a sexual assault prevention program as part of a new student orientation. A brief discussion of the handling of missing data is found in the analysis section of this paper.

While the sexual assault prevention program is offered to all incoming freshman, only those students living in on-campus housing are required to participate in the program. All students living in specified first-year halls and affiliated with one of the coeducational, undergraduate colleges at this university were included in the study, which represented 81.4 percent of the total population of students living in residence halls on campus. Table 1 contains demographic information for the sample. Thirty-four percent of the respondents had attended a sexual assault prevention program before and thirty-five percent knew someone who had been sexually assaulted. Given the increased incidence of sexual assaults among the nation's teenage population and the increased attention to prevention within our public schools (Hilton, Harris, Rice, Krans, & Lavigne, 1998), it is not surprising that about one-third of the sample have experience with both sexual assault and prevention programs.

Measures

The Scale for the Identification of Acquaintance Rape Attitudes was designed to measure attitudes about acquaintance rape, including indi-

TABLE 1. Sample Descriptive Information

$N = 1,782^+$

Gender	Male	880
	Female	902
Ethnicity	White	55%
	Asian/Pacific Islander	25%
	Black	6%
	Mexican American/Hispanic	6%
	Multiracial	3%
	American Indian/Alaskan Native	<1%
Age	Mean	17.66
	SD	0.57
Athlete (Participating in intercollegiate, NCAA sports)		12%
Intending to pledge a fraternity/sorority		6%
First in family to attend college		28%
Previously attended a sexual assault program		34%
Know someone who was sexually assaulted		35%

[+]Note: the sample size before listwise deletion was 2,163.

vidual beliefs about dating, sex, and rape (Humphrey & Hillenbrand-Gunn, 1996). The scale is comprised of thirty-three items rated on a six-point Likert scale ranging from (0) strongly disagree to (5) strongly agree. Examples of the individual items are: "After a woman agrees to have sexual intercourse, it is OK for her to change her mind"; "Any time a woman dresses seductively, she is indicating that she is willing to have sexual intercourse"; and "When women claim they were raped, it is usually because they have regrets about letting sexual activity go too far." High scores indicate that the respondent is expressing attitudes that are supportive of sexual assault.

Administration Procedures

The Scale for the Identification of Acquaintance Rape Attitudes was distributed to students a total of three times: prior to the sexual assault prevention program, immediately after participation in the program, and then three months later. Data from the initial pretest was utilized in this study. The pretest was administered on the first day of the semester. Students were guaranteed confidentiality in the directions read by the residence hall staff and again in the informed consent form.

Analysis Strategy

Confirmatory Factor Analysis (CFA). The confirmatory factor analysis addressed the following research question: Can this sample provide support for the unidimensionality of the Scale for the Identification of Acquaintance Rape Attitudes' assessment of acquaintance rape attitudes?

In order to address issues related to missing data and the non-normal distribution of the data, various model estimation strategies were performed. Non-normal distribution of data was addressed by using robust statistics associated with the Maximum Likelihood (ML) estimation of the CFA models, for example Satorra-Bentler Scaled Chi-Squared statistic (S-B X^2), Robust CFI and robust standard errors (Bentler, 1995; Bentler & Dijkstra, 1985; Satorra & Bentler,1988ab). Maximum Likelihood estimates with robust statistics were conducted with EQS 5.7b (Bentler, 1995). Research indicates that robust statistics associated with ML are the most efficient method, except in those studies that involve very large sample sizes (West, Finch, & Curran, 1995). In cases involving very large sample sizes Asymptotically Distribution Free (ADF) estimation is as efficient as ML with robust test statistics (West, Finch, & Curran, 1995). Addressing issues related to missing data were addressed by using Full Information Maximum Likelihood estimation (FIML; Arbuckle & Wothke, 1999). Full Information Maximum Likelihood estimates were performed by using AMOS 4.0 (Arbuckle & Wothke, 1999). A brief discussion of the procedures for handling missing data will be addressed in the next section.

Missing data procedures. The missing data analysis proceeded in three stages: (1) Examination of the study sample's demographics; (2) Examination of the amount and pattern of missing survey items, and lastly, (3) Examination of the stability of findings when estimated using two estimation methods. Maximum Likelihood (ML) with Satorra-Bentler Scaled Chi-Square and robust standard errors (Satorra & Bentler, 1994) was compared to Full Information Maximum Likelihood estimates (FIML; Arbuckle & Wothke, 1999). Listwise deletion of missing data was used for the ML estimate and no cases were deleted for the FIML estimate.

Considering the difficulty involved in determining the response mechanism underlying missing data in a study, demographics of the study's sample and the pattern of missing data were examined to provide some insight into the possibility that data in this study was either "missing completely at random" (MCAR) or "missing at random"

(MAR). Full Information Maximum Likelihood estimates provide efficient parameter estimates in both situations (Enders & Bandalos, 2001). Following the recommendations of Pigott (2001), the sensitivity of results to different assumptions about the response mechanism was compared. This was done by comparing the sensitivity of results based on complete cases (i.e., ML with robust statistics estimate) to model-based methods for multivariate normal missing data (i.e., FIML estimate).

Model evaluation. Following the recommendation of Bentler (2000), Hu and Bentler (1999), and Mulaik and Millsap (2000), the Comparative Fit Index (CFI) and the Root Mean Squared Error of Approximation (RMSEA) were used to evaluate the quality of the model fit. Confirmatory factor analysis models were evaluated as having a good fit when the CFI is greater than or equal to .95 and the RMSEA is less than or equal to .06 (Hu & Bentler, 1999). Additionally, the model Chi-Square is presented along with the Relative Chi-Square (χ^2/df). Given the sensitivity of Chi-Square to sample size (e.g., Bentler, 1995; Kline, 1998) and questions regarding the value of the relative Chi-Square (e.g., Wheaton, 1987), the CFI and RMSEA were given greater weight when evaluating model fit. Following the recommendations of Carmines and McIver (1981) and Kline (1998), a relative Chi-Square less than or equal to 3 indicates a good fitting model.

Multi-group factorial and mean-structure analysis. Research has consistently indicated distinctions between male and female attitudes toward sexual assault and harassment (Anderson, Cooper, & Okamura, 1997). Therefore, the potential differences between male and female attitudes toward acquaintance rape were examined. As the SIARA aims to measure attitudes towards acquaintance rape, its contents and applicability should be equally relevant for qualitatively different groups such as males and females. Thus, the second research question focused on the potential factorial and mean structure invariance of the SIARA across gender.

The testing of factorial invariance has long been recommended as a means to determine comparative validity across groups (Bentler, 1995; Bentler & Dudgeon, 1996; Jöreskog, 1971, 1993). Confirmatory factor analysis multi-group comparison analysis was used to examine the potential invariance of the measurement model and the latent mean structure between males and females (Bentler, 1980; Byrne, Shavelson, & Muthen, 1989). Using EQS 5.7b, the equality of the factor loadings and the latent means for the common measurement model between males and females were tested using the Lagrange Multiplier Test (LM Test). The LM test is the recommended procedure to test the appropriateness of cross sample constraints, e.g., equality of factor loadings and latent means across samples (Bentler, 1995; Byrne, 1994; Hu & Bentler, 1995; Jöreskog, 1993). The LM test assesses equality constraints multivariately. The analysis unfolds in two phases: (1) preliminary single-group analyses and (2) fitting the multi-group model.

The preliminary single-group analysis involved establishing the baseline model for each group separately. This model represents the one that best fits the data. The second phase involved the estimation of each group's base model simultaneously with equivalence constraints imposed between the two samples. Equivalency constraints for all factor loadings, covariances between the two factors and parameters associated with the mean structure, will be imposed. For model identification purposes the factor intercepts for the female group were set to zero; therefore, the female sample operates as a reference group against which latent means for the male sample are compared. A detailed discussion of identification with multi-group latent means structure models can be found in Byrne (1994). The fit of the multi-group model with equivalence constraints was evaluated by examining the CFI and the LM tests of the equality of the models constraints (Bentler, 1995; Byrne, 1994).

RESULTS

Missing Data Analysis

Demographically the study's sample did not differ significantly from the target population as it relates to gender, ethnicity or age. Additionally, there were no significant differences in the response rate across resident halls. Overall, the percentage of missing item level data ranged from 2 to 3 percent. Those participants with completed survey data did not differ descriptively from those who did not have complete survey data. Finally, the confirmatory factor analysis results were consistent across estimation techniques, therefore, the ML with listwise deletion for missing data results will be presented.

Item Analysis

In order to conserve space, the zero-order correlation matrixes were not included in this article. These tables are available upon request from the authors. Figure 1 displays the distribution of the SIARA scale composite scores for male and female subjects. Summing the thirty-three items on the SIARA created the composite scores. High scores indicate that the individual expressed attitudes that were supportive of sexual assault, i.e., they expressed attitudes that endorsed rape myths (Humphrey & Hillenbrand-Gunn, 1996). Theoretically the scores could range from zero to one hundred and sixty-five. In the sample the scores ranged from five to one hundred and fifty-five. Visual inspection of the distribution of the composite scores for males and females separately (i.e., inspection of boxplots and normal probability plots), along with statistical tests of normality (i.e., Shapiro-Wilks & Kolmogorov-Smirnov Lilliefors statistics) indicate a slight degree of positive skewness in the distribution of scores.

Confirmatory Factor Analysis Results

Table 2 contains the model fit information for the various models examined. The one factor model did not provide an adequate fit for any of the sample conditions (i.e., males, females, or overall); both the Robust

FIGURE 1. Distribution SIARA Scale Composite Scores by Gender. The Composite Score Was Based on the Summation of Thirty-Three Scale Items.

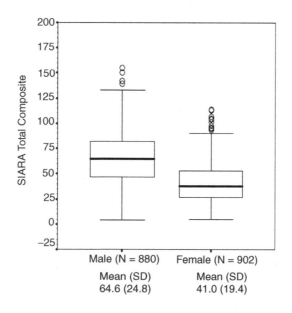

TABLE 2. Goodness-of-Fit Indices for the CFA Models

Overall Sample (N = 1,782)

Model	df	S-B χ^2	S-B χ^2/df	RCFI	AGFI	RMSEA (90% CI)
One Factor	495	3,227	6.5	0.84	0.81	0.068 (0.066, 0.070)
Two Factor Model (Sexual Expectations & Rape Mythology)	88	386	4.4	0.95	0.96	0.048 (0.044, 0.052)

Males (N = 880)

Model	df	S-B χ^2	S-B χ^2/df	RCFI	AGFI	RMSEA (90% CI)
One Factor	495	2,538	5.1	0.78	0.77	0.076 (0.073, 0.078)
Two Factor Model (Sexual Expectations & Rape Mythology)	88	258	2.9	0.95	0.95	0.053 (0.047, 0.059)

Female (N = 902)

Model	df	S-B χ^2	S-B χ^2/df	RCFI	AGFI	RMSEA (90% CI)
One Factor	495	3,212	6.5	0.61	0.74	0.087 (0.084, 0.089)
Two Factor Model (Sexual Expectations & Rape Mythology)	88	233	2.6	0.95	0.96	0.051 (0.045, 0.058)

S-B χ^2 = Satorra-Bentler Scaled Chi-Square; S-B χ^2/df = Relative Chi-Square; RCFI = Robust Comparative Fit Index; AGFI = Adjusted Goodness-of-Fit Index; RMSEA = Root Mean Error of Approximation; 90% CI = 90% confidence interval.
One factor model includes the original 33 items.
Two factor model = Sexual Expectations & Rape Mythology

CFI and Adjusted Goodness-of-Fit Index (AGFI) were below .95, RMSEA were above .06 and relative chi-squares were above three. It should be noted that, in an attempt to improve the fit of the one factor models, the correlation among various error terms was examined such as the correlation among items that focused on women's behavior and those focusing on men's behavior. Given that the use of parameter chance statistics (e.g., LM and Wald Test) as the sole guide to the respecification of the CFA model could lead to a new model that capitalizes on chance and has no theoretical meaningfulness (Bentler, 2000; Byrne, 1994), the researchers used Anderson, Cooper, and Okamura's (1997) meta-analysis of gender differences in attitudes towards rape to assist in the respecification process.

Anderson, Cooper, and Okamura (1997) noted that attitudes toward rape could be divided into four dimensions: attitudinal, behavioral, experiential and personality. Considering the face validity of the SIARA's thirty-three items, it appears that only the attitudinal and behavioral dimensions of rape attitudes are addressed. Fourteen of the items addressed the attitudinal dimension and nineteen of the items addressed the behavioral dimension. The CFA for this two-factor model and review of parameter change statistics (e.g., LM and Wald Test) resulted in the dropping of nineteen items because they did not significantly load on either of the two factors nor did they appear to create any meaningful additional factors. As a result, the two-factor model contained six items consistent with a sexual expectation dimension and eight items consistent with a rape mythology dimension (see Table 3). Figures 2 and 3 display the distribution of the composite scores for the two factors for

TABLE 3. Scale Items

Sexual expectations items

1. When a woman passionately kisses her date, she is letting him know that she wants to have sexual intercourse.

2. If a woman does not physically resist a man's sexual advances, it is safe for the man to assume that the woman wants to have sexual intercourse.

3. If a woman goes to her date's apartment, she is letting her date know that she is open to having sexual intercourse.

4. Any time a woman dresses seductively, she is indicating that she is willing to have sexual intercourse.

5. If a woman initiates physical contact on a date, it is OK for her partner to assume she wants to have sexual intercourse.

6. If a woman is saying "yes" to sexual intercourse with her body language, but she is saying "no" verbally, a man should listen to the woman's body language because it is more accurate.

Rape mythology items

1. A person who thinks all sexual jokes about women are offensive is just overreacting.

2. The extent of acquaintance rape on college campuses has been greatly exaggerated.

3. It is not right for a man to be accused of raping his date if the date does not say "no" to sexual intercourse.

4. It is OK for a man to joke around with his friends about forcing a woman to have sexual intercourse, as long as he never actually does it.

5. When an unattractive woman is raped, it can be assumed that she did more to provoke it than an attractive woman would.

6. When rape happens on a date, it is usually because the woman sends mixed messages to the man about what she wants sexually.

7. A woman who gets upset when a man jokingly grabs her breast at a party is overreacting.

8. A woman would probably think it was romantic if a man assumed she wanted to have sexual intercourse without actually asking her first.

FIGURE 2. Distribution Sexual Expectation Scale Composite Scores by Gender. The Composite Score Was Based on the Summation of Six Items.

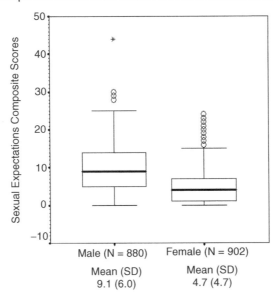

males and females. Table 2 has the fit information for the two-factor model (e.g., sexual expectations and rape mythology). Tables 4 and 5 present the factor loadings and robust standard errors for the two-factor model. Fit indices for the two-factor model were adequate, while the relative chi-square exceeded 3.0 for the overall sample; the RMSEA, RCFI and AGFI for all samples were within acceptable ranges.

Factorial Invariance and Mean Structure Analysis

Factorial invariance. The fit statistics for the multi-group CFA model had equivalency constraints between males and females for all factor loadings. Given the overly restrictive nature of the global test of the equality of covariance structure across the two groups and tests of equality that involve error variances and covariance, only the invariance of factor loadings was tested (Byrne, 2001). The fit statistics for the multi-group model that had equivalency constraints for all the factor loadings are $\chi^2 = 416$, $df = 139$, p < .001; $\chi^2/df = 3.0$; CFI = .95. In reviewing the LM χ^2 multivariate statistics, however, five constraints ap-

FIGURE 3. Distribution Rape Myth Scale Composite Scores by Gender. The Composite Score Was Based on the Summation of Eight Items.

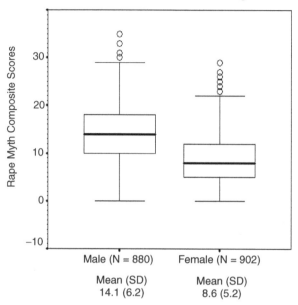

peared to be misspecified, but their release did not significantly improve the model fit. While the change in chi-square was significant between the two nested models ($\Delta\chi^2 = 13$, $df = 6$, p = .04), the CFI for the respecified model was not meaningfully different from the one found in the model with all of the original equivalency constraints. When rounded, both fit indexes (i.e., CFI and AGFI) were 0.95.

Mean structure analysis. The goodness-of-fit statistics show for the mean-structure model a good fit to the multi-group data, as indicated by a CFI of 0.95. In reviewing the LM χ^2 multivariate statistics, eight constraints appeared to be misspecified, but their release did not appear to significantly improve the model fit. While the change in χ^2 was significant between the two nested models ($\Delta\chi^2 = 34$, $df = 5$, p < .001), the CFI for the respecified model was not meaningfully different from the one found in the model with all of the original equivalency constraints. When rounded, both fit indexes (i.e., CFI and AGFI) were 0.95.

Summary of findings. The two-factor model fit the sample of students well. The two dimensions in that model are Sexual Expectations and Rape Mythology. Additionally, the data did not provide evidence that

TABLE 4A. *Standardized Solutions by Confirmatory Factor Analysis for the Two-Factor Model. Factor Loadings and Robust Standard Errors

Male
(N = 880)

Item	Factors	
	Sexual Expectations	
	Factor Loading (SE)	R^2
1. When a woman passionately kisses her date, she is letting him know that she wants to have sexual intercourse.	.69 (---)	.48
2. If a woman does not physically resist a man's sexual advances, it is safe for the man to assume that the woman wants to have sexual intercourse.	.62 (.11)	.38
3. If a woman goes to her date's apartment, she is letting her date know that she is open to having sexual intercourse.	.71 (.04)	.52
4. Any time a woman dresses seductively, she is indicating that she is willing to have sexual intercourse.	.72 (.06)	.53
5. If a woman initiates physical contact on a date, it is OK for her partner to assume she wants to have sexual intercourse.	.62 (.06)	.38
6. If a woman is saying "yes" to sexual intercourse with her body language, but she is saying "no" verbally, a man should listen to the woman's body language because it is more accurate.	.53 (.06)	.28

Note. (–) = Factor fixed to 1.0 for model identification purposes and the standard error was not estimated.
*Standardized Factor loading (standard error), all factor loadings are significant at the .05 level. CFAs were conducted with EQS 5.7b using maximum likelihood (ML) estimates derived from covariance matrixes based on listwise deletion for missing data.

there were any differences in the factor loadings or latent mean structure of the model for male and female students.

DISCUSSION

The emergence of two factors, Sexual Expectations and Rape Mythology, offers important insight into the structure of attitudes about acquaintance rape for late adolescent youth attending college in this sample. Both factors build upon the existing theoretical foundations for examining attitudes about rape but apply these frameworks specifically to the issue of acquaintance rape. The factors were consistent for males and females, which indicates a similar structure of attitudes for both genders. The Rape Mythology factor is theoretically consistent with

TABLE 4B. *Standardized Solutions by Confirmatory Factor Analysis for the Two-Factor Model. Factor Loadings and Robust Standard Errors

Male
($N = 880$)

Item	Factor	
	Rape Mythology	
	Factor Loading (SE)	R^2
1. A person who thinks all sexual jokes about women are offensive is just overreacting.	.46 (--)	.21
2. The extent of acquaintance rape on college campuses has been greatly exaggerated.	.50 (.08)	.25
3. It is not right for a man to be accused of raping his date if the date does not say "no" to sexual intercourse.	.44 (.10)	.21
4. It is OK for a man to joke around with his friends about forcing a woman to have sexual intercourse, as long as he never actually does it.	.73 (.10)	.26
5. When an unattractive woman is raped, it can be assumed that she did more to provoke it than an attractive woman would.	.61 (.11)	.37
6. When rape happens on a date, it is usually because the woman sends mixed messages to the man about what she wants sexually.	.62 (.10)	.40
7. A woman who gets upset when a man jokingly grabs her breast at a party is overreacting.	.60 (.09)	.35
8. A woman would probably think it was romantic if a man assumed she wanted to have sexual intercourse without actually asking her first.	.65 (.10)	.41

Note. (–) = Factor fixed to 1.0 for model identification purposes and the standard error was not estimated.
*Standardized Factor Loading (standard error), all factor loadings are significant at the .05 level.
Factor loadings and robust standard errors for the covariance between the two factors: = .84 (.05).
Factor loadings and robust standard errors for the covariance between the error terms for Q1 and Q4 =.19 (.06).
S-B χ^2= 258; df = 88; p < .05; Robust Comparative Fit Index =. 95; Goodness-of-Fit Index = .95; RMSEA = 0.053, 95% CI (0.047, 0.059).

previous literature that supports the existence of prejudicial beliefs about rape, rape victims, and perpetrators (Burt, 1980). The items for this factor questioned the truthfulness of victims, incidence, and severity of harassment and rape on campus. The acknowledgement of the above-mentioned items suggests that there exist certain myths about acquaintance rape that continue to shape the social interactions among late adolescent college students.

TABLE 5A. *Standardized Solutions by Confirmatory Factor Analysis for the Two-Factor Model. Factor Loadings and Robust Standard Errors

Female
(N = 902)

Item	Factors	
	Sexual Expectations	
	Factor Loading (SE)	R^2
1. When a woman passionately kisses her date, she is letting him know that she wants to have sexual intercourse.	.58 (---)	.34
2. If a woman does not physically resist a man's sexual advances, it is safe for the man to assume that the woman wants to have sexual intercourse.	.55 (.10)	.30
3. If a woman goes to her date's apartment, she is letting her date know that she is open to having sexual intercourse.	.63 (.08)	.40
4. Any time a woman dresses seductively, she is indicating that she is willing to have sexual intercourse.	.61 (.05)	.37
5. If a woman initiates physical contact on a date, it is OK for her partner to assume she wants to have sexual intercourse.	.73 (.08)	.53
6. If a woman is saying "yes" to sexual intercourse with her body language, but she is saying "no" verbally, a man should listen to the woman's body language because it is more accurate.	.41 (.05)	.16

Note. (–) = Factor fixed to 1.0 for model identification purposes and the standard error was not estimated.
*Standardized Factor Loading (standard error), all factor loadings are significant at the .05 level. CFAs were conducted with EQS 5.7b using maximum likelihood (ML) estimates derived from covariance matrixes based on listwise deletion for missing data.

Prevention programs' attention to the various rape myths that continue to shape the social development of late adolescence youth as they move into adulthood appears to be appropriate. Further exploration may reveal that programming should address rape as part of a spectrum of violence and emphasize the impact that various forms of violence may have on victims' social development and the quality of their ability to freely experience college life.

The presence of the Sexual Expectations factor reflects gendered-based social scripts that direct the interactions among young adults. All of the items on this factor reflect perceptions about a woman's willingness to have sex based on her behaviors. It is similar to Burt's (1980) Victim Responsibility factor, which referred to items that held a woman

TABLE 5B. *Standardized Solutions by Confirmatory Factor Analysis for the Two-Factor Model. Factor Loadings and Robust Standard Errors

Female (N = 902)		
Item	Factor	
	Rape Mythology	
	Factor Loading (SE)	R^2
1. A person who thinks all sexual jokes about women are offensive is just overreacting.	.48 (---)	.22
2. The extent of acquaintance rape on college campuses has been greatly exaggerated.	.42 (.08)	.18
3. It is not right for a man to be accused of raping his date if the date does not say "no" to sexual intercourse.	.37 (.10)	.14
4. It is OK for a man to joke around with his friends about forcing a woman to have sexual intercourse, as long as he never actually does it.	.46 (.08)	.17
5. When an unattractive woman is raped, it can be assumed that she did more to provoke it than an attractive woman would.	.53 (.08)	.29
6. When rape happens on a date it is usually because the woman sends mixed messages to the man about what she wants sexually.	.57 (.09)	.35
7. A woman who gets upset when a man jokingly grabs her breast at a party is overreacting.	.45 (.07)	.19
8. A woman would probably think it was romantic if a man assumed she wanted to have sexual intercourse without actually asking her first.	.56 (.08)	.29

Note. (–) = Factor fixed to 1.0 for model identification purposes and the standard error was not estimated.
*Standardized Factor Loading (standard error), all factor loadings are significant at the .05 level.
Factor loadings and robust standard errors for the covariance between the two factors: .80 (.05).
Factor loadings and robust standard errors for the covariance between the error terms for Q1 and Q4: .20 (.06).
S-B χ^2 = 233; df = 88; $p < .05$; Robust Comparative Fit Index =. 95; Goodness-of-Fit Index = .96; RMSEA = 0.053, 95% CI (0.047, 0.059).

responsible for sexual victimization. Sexual Expectations can be distinguished from Burt's (1980) Victim Responsibility factor in that it represents items particular to acquaintance rape. The Sexual Expectations factor is important to consider when designing appropriate interventions for late adolescent youth as they progress in their development of adult intimate relationships.

This study illuminates a set of limitations with the SIARA's ability to accurately assess a range of students' attitudes about dating, sexual expectations, and rape. For both male and female respondents, the distribution of scores was slightly positively skewed. This indicates that either many students have adopted socially appropriate attitudes toward acquaintance rape and/or there is a response bias present. Assuming the latter, the biased results of this study suggest some revisions for future development of instruments to more accurately measure student attitudes about issues of sexual assault.

Perhaps most significantly, the distribution of responses to the SIARA suggests that the effects of social desirability need to be further examined. For a serious issue like sexual assault, students may feel pressured to give the politically or socially "correct" answer rather than what they truly feel. This raises questions about both the administration and design of the instrument. The fact that the students in this study knew that the SIARA was being administered through the Department of Sexual Assault Services may have increased their likelihood to provide socially desirable responses. The Department of Sexual Assault Services' involvement with the survey was clearly conveyed to each respondent at the time the survey was distributed and also their name appeared on the cover letter. Perhaps administration from a more "neutral" source would be beneficial.

In addition to changing the process of distributing the survey, tools could be used to assess the true impact of social desirability upon responses. The issue of social desirability has been extensively examined by several researchers (e.g., Crowne & Marlowe, 1964; Paulhus, 1984) and applied to the measurement of similarly sensitive issues such as intimate violence (Sugarman & Hotaling, 1997); HIV (Latkin & Vlahov, 1998); and sexuality (Meston et al., 1998). Researchers have recognized the impact of social desirability and have accounted for this in the design of their instruments through the employment of mechanisms such as the use of lie scales (Abramson, 1973) or measure of social desirability (Crowne & Marlowe, 1964). The social desirability research should be consulted when devising future sexual assault measurement instruments to build in appropriate tests for social desirability so that the results reflect greater accuracy.

Second, the need for a guarantee of anonymity for respondents is emphasized by these results. While the administration of this survey included explicit statements that students would remain anonymous, they were still required to sign an informed consent form and provide the last four digits of their Social Security numbers. While they were told that these numbers would only allow for the linking of their responses across the three waves of this study, perhaps the submission of even the slightest self-identifying information caused suspicion by respondents and therefore biased responses. This suggests that the request for demographic information and any other self-identifying information should be kept to an absolute minimum. For the purposes of matching pre-tests and post-tests, perhaps students can be given a random number or some other meaningless code. Identifying information could be eliminated entirely if the change in groups, rather than in individuals, was measured. Informed consent is a more problematic issue but perhaps more creative means can be explored.

This study indicates that the SIARA is a useful outcome measure for assessing the impact of sexual assault prevention programming on changing attitudes about sexual expectations and rape mythology for this sample. Replication of these results with other samples is crucial for determining its utility as an evaluation tool for measuring these factors. If further testing confirms the presence of these factors, the SIARA could be revised to contain fourteen items rather than thirty-three. Further exploration of these factors may be useful in developing appropriate prevention programming and the measurement of its impact.

REFERENCES

Abel, E. M. (2001). Comparing the social service utilization, exposure to violence, and trauma symptomology of domestic violence female "victims" and female "batterers." *Journal of Family Violence, 16*(4), 401-420.

Abramson, P. R. (1973). The relationship of the frequency of masturbation to several aspects of personality and behavior. *The Journal of Sex Research, 9,* 132-142.

Ackard, D. M., & Neumark-Sztainer, D. (2002). Date violence and date rape among adolescents: Associations with disordered eating behaviors and psychological health. *Child Abuse & Neglect, 26*(5), 455-473.

Ambuel, B., Butler, D., Hamberger, L. K., Lawrence, S., & Guse, C. (2003). Female and male medical students' exposure to violence: Impact on well-being and perceived capacity to help battered women. *Journal of Comparative Family Studies, 34*(1), 113-135.

Anderson, K. B., Cooper, H., & Okamura, L. (1997). Individual differences and attitudes toward rape: A meta-analytic review. *Personality and Social Psychology Bulletin, 23*(3), 295-315.

Arbuckle, J. L., & Wothke, W. (1999). *Amos 4.0 user's guide.* Chicago, IL: Small Waters Corporation.

Bentler, P. M., & Dijkstra, T. (1985). Efficient estimation via linearization in structural models. In P. R. Krishnaiah (Ed.), *Multivariate analysis VI* (pp. 9-42). Amsterdam: North-Holland.

Bentler, P. M. (1980). Multivariate analysis with latent variables: Causal modeling. *Annual Review of Psychology, 21,* 419-456.

Bentler, P. M. (1995). *EQS: Structural equation program manual.* Los Angeles: Multivariate Software, Inc.

Bentler, P. M. (2000). Rites, wrongs, and gold in model testing. *Structural Equation Modeling, 7*(1), 82-91.

Bentler, P. M., & Dudgeon, P. (1996). Covariance structure analysis: Statistical practice, theory, and directions. *Annual Review of Psychology, 47,* 563-592.

Black, B., Weisz, A., Coats, S., & Patterson, D. (2000). Evaluating a psychoeducational sexual assault prevention program incorporating theatrical presentation, peer education, and social work. *Research on Social Work Practice, 10*(5), 589-606.

Burt, M. (1980). Cultural myths and support for rape. *Journal of Personality & Social Psychology, 2,* 217-230.

Byrne, B. M., Shavelson, R. J., & Muthen, B. (1989). Testing the equivalence of factor covariance and mean structures: The issues of partial measurement invariance. *Psychological Bulletin, 105,* 456-466.

Byrne, B. M. (1994). *Structural equation modeling with EQS and EQS/Windows: Basic concepts, applications, and programming.* Thousands Oaks, CA: Sage Publications.

Byrne, B. M. (2001). *Structural equation modeling with AMOS: Basic concepts, applications and programming.* Mahwah, NJ: Lawrence Erlbaum Associates.

Carmines, E. G., & McIver, J. P. (1981). Analyzing models with unobserved variables. In G. W. Bohrnstedt & E. F. Borgatta (Eds.), *Social measurement: Current issues* (p. 80). Beverly Hills: Sage Publications.

Cowan, C. P., Lee, C., Levy, D., & Snyder, D. (1988). Dominance and inequality in X-rated videocassettes. *Psychology of Women Quarterly, 12*(3), 299-311.

Crowne, D. P., & Marlowe, D. A. (1964). *The approval motive.* New York, NY: Wiley.

Danis, F. S. (2003). The criminalization of domestic violence: What social workers need to know. *Social Work, 48*(2), 237-246.

Earle, J. P. (1996). Acquaintance rape workshops: Their effectiveness in changing the attitudes of first year college men. *NASPA Journal, 34,* 1-16.

Enders, C. K., & Bandalos, D. L. (2001). The relative performance of full information maximum likelihood estimation for missing data in structural equation models. *Structural Equation Modeling, 8*(3), 430-457.

Fisher, R. S., Cullen, F. T., & Turner, M. G. (2000). *The sexual victimization of college women (NCJ 182369).* Washington, DC: U.S. Department of Justice.

Gender and Health Unit (2003). Gender-based violence: A public health and human rights problem, In *Violence against women: The health sector's response* (pp. 4-7). Annapolis, MD: Pan American Health Organization.

Guttman, H. A. (2002). The epigenesis of the family system as a context for individual development. *Family Process, 41*(3), 533-545.

Hilton, N. Z., Harris, G. T., Rice, M. E., Krans, T. S., & Lavigne, S. E. (1998). Antiviolence education in high schools: Implementation and evaluation. *Journal of Interpersonal Violence, 13*(6), 726-742.

Hinck, S. S., & Thomas, R. W. (1999). Rape myth acceptance in college students: How far have we come? *Sex Roles, 40*(9-10), 815-832.

Hines, D. A., & Saudino, K. J. (2002). Intergenerational transmission of intimate partner violence: A behavioral genetic perspective. *Trauma Violence & Abuse, 3*(3), 210-225.

Holcomb, D. R., Savage, M. P., Seehafer, R., & Waalkes, D. M. (2002). A mixed-gender date rape prevention intervention targeting freshman-college athletes. *College Student Journal, 36*(2), 165-180.

Holcomb, D. R., Sarvela, P. D., Sondag, K. A., & Holcomb, L. C. (1993). An evaluation of a mixed-gender date rape prevention workshop. *Journal of American College Health, 41*, 159-164.

Hu, L.-T., & Bentler, P. M. (1999). Cutoff criteria for fit indexes in covariance structure analysis: Conventional criteria versus new alternatives. *Structural Equation Modeling, 6*, 1-56.

Humphreys, C., & Thiara, R. (2003). Mental health and domestic violence: 'I call it symptoms of abuse.' *The British Journal of Social Work, 33*(2), 209-226.

Jimenez, J. A., & Abreu, J. M. (2003). Race and sex effects on attitudinal perceptions of acquaintance rape. *Journal of Counseling Psychology, 50*(2), 252-256.

Jöreskog, K. (1971). Simultaneous factor analysis in several populations. *Psychometrika, 36*, 409-426.

Jöreskog, K. (1993). Testing structural equation models. In K. A. Bollen & J. S. Long (Eds.), *Testing structural equation models* (pp. 294-316). Newbury Park, CA: Sage Publications.

Jöreskog, K. G. (1971). Simultaneous factor analysis in several populations. *Psychometrika, 36*, 409-426.

Kline, R. B. (1998). *Principles and practices of structural equation modeling.* New York: Guilford Press.

Latkin, C. A., & Vlahov, D. (1998). Socially desirable response tendency as a correlate of accuracy of self-reported HIV serostatus for HIV seropositive injection drug users. *Addiction, 93*, 1191-1197.

Lonsway, K.A., & Fitzgerald, L.F. (1984). Rape myths in review. *Psychology of Women Quarterly, 18*(2),133-164.

Lonsway, K. A., & Kothari, C. (2000). First year campus acquaintance rape education: Evaluating the impact of a mandatory intervention. *Psychology of Women Quarterly, 24*(3), 220-232.

Meston, C. M., Heiman, J.R., Trapnell, P. D., & Paulhus, D. L. (1998). Socially desirable responding and sexual self-reports. *The Journal of Sex Research, 35* (2), 148- 157.

Muehlenhard, C. L., & Rodgers, C. S. (1998). Token resistance to sex: New perspectives on an old stereotype. *Psychology of Women Quarterly, 22*(3), 443-463.

Mulaik, S. A., & Millsap, R. E. (2000). Doing the four-step right. *Structural Equation Modeling, 7*(1), 36-73.

Paulhus, D. L. (1984). Two-component models of socially desirability responding. *Journal of Personality &Social Psychology, 46*, 598-609.

Payne, D. L., Lonsway, K. A., & Fitzgerald, L. F. (1999). Rape myth acceptance: Exploration of its structure and its measurement using the Illinois Rape Myth Acceptance Scale. *Journal of Research in Personality, 33*(1), 27-68.

Pigott, T. D. (2001). A review of methods for missing data. *Educational Research & Evaluation, 7*(4), 353.

Rand, M. R., & Saltzman, L. E. (2003). The nature and extent of recurring intimate partner violence against women in the United States. *Journal of Comparative Family Studies, 34*(1), 137-149.

Satorra, A., & Bentler, P. M. (1994). Corrections to test statistics and standard errors in covariance structure analysis. In A. V. Eye & C. C. Clogg (Eds.), *Latent variables analysis: Applications for developmental research* (pp. 399-419). Thousand Oaks, CA: Sage.

Schaeffer, A. M., &Nelson, E. (1993). Rape-supportive attitudes: Effects of on-campus residence and education. *Journal of College Student Development, 34*(3), 175-179.

Sugarman, D. B., & Hotaling, G. T. (1997). Intimate violence and social desirability: A meta-analytic review. *Journal of Interpersonal Violence, 12*(2), 275-290.

Tjaden, P., & Thoennes, N. (2000). *Full report of the prevalence, incidence, and consequences of violence against women* (Report No. NCJ 183781). Washington, DC: National Institute of Justice and Center for Disease Control and Prevention.

Tolan, P. H., Gorman-Smith, D., & Henry, D. B. (2003). The developmental ecology of urban males' youth violence. *Developmental Psychology, 39*(2), 274-291.

Venis, S., & Horton, R. (2002). Violence against women: A global burden. *Lancet, 359* (9313), 1172.

West, S. G., Finch, J. F., & Curran, P. J. (1995). Structural equation models with nonnormal variables: Problems and remedies. In R. H. Hoyle (Ed.), *Structural equation modeling: Concepts, issues and applications* (pp. 56-75). Thousand Oaks, CA: Sage Publications.

Wheaton, B. (1987). Assessment of fit in over-identified models with latent variables. *Sociological Methods and Research, 16,* 118-154.

Wood, J. M., Tatryn, D. J., & Gorsuch, R. L. (1996). Effects of under- and over-extraction on principal axis factor analysis with varimax rotation. *Psychological Methods, 1,* 354-365.

Index

T - #0514 - 101024 - C0 - 212/152/14 - PB - 9780789030832 - Gloss Lamination